The Anti-Medicine

Eating to Live Without Disease

PART 2

by Albert Mosséri

INDEX

- CHAPTER 1: Salt is a Killer 03
- CHAPTER 2: No Bread, No Grains 16
- CHAPTER 3: Did Humans Adapt to Eat Meat and Bread? 20
- CHAPTER 4: Can We Enjoy Meat? 26
- CHAPTER 5: Can We Develop a Tolerance to Wine, Coffee, and Anxiolytics? 28
- CHAPTER 6: The Paradise Diet, According to Dr. Lovewisdom 34
- CHAPTER 7: How to Find Your Way Among Various Dietary Systems 47
- CHAPTER 8: Table Of Comparative Anatomy And Physiology ... 52
- CHAPTER 9: Comparative Anatomy And Physiology 54
- CHAPTER 10: Testimonials 71

CHAPTER 1: Salt is a Killer

On July 7, 1970, the *TASS Russian News Agency* sent a telegram containing the following news, entitled "Salt is a Killer," from Moscow to its correspondents worldwide. The Post and Times—Star (Cincinnati), an American Newspaper quoted in the Hygienic Review, describes the news as follows:

"Soviet researchers have labeled salt as a dangerous killer which, when abused, has the power to cause cardiac, hepatic, renal and stomach disease. This assessment is evidenced in research carried out by researchers at the Institute of Therapeutics and Experimental Pathology in Sukhumi.

"According to the TASS Russian News Agency, the Soviet researchers conducted experiments on baboons and studied the health of people living in regions where the water is high in sodium, such as Ukraine, Japan, Canada, Czechoslovakia and the Bahamas.

"From these studies, they concluded that high concentrations of salt could lead to dangerous disturbances in all human organ systems." – Hygienic Review.

It's been more than 100 years since Natural Hygiene practitioners, led by Sylvester Graham and Dr. Russel T. Trall, proved beyond a shadow of a doubt that salt is harmful.

"These jokers that the TASS Russian News Agency is calling researchers," says Shelton, "have always insisted that salt is useful for human beings. These very same jokers who, today, are labeling salt as a killer!"

However, this is always the case in medicine. We discover a medication, and people say that it works miracles; then, it's found out that the drug has severe side effects and that it can kill the people it means to help. Nevertheless, the drug is defended just long enough for another drug to be found in an infinite, endless loop, always profiting the pharmaceutical manufacturers whose stocks never stop growing.

Furthermore, naturopaths, ignorant and always lagging behind modern medicine, continue to advocate using salt in moderation. They have yet to catch up with these Russian doctors.

If you tell someone to eat salt in moderation, I'll bet you that they'll continue to eat it as they always have without decreasing their consumption in the slightest. However, if you tell the same person to eliminate salt from their diet, they will only occasionally eat it and in small quantities.

In reality, salt is a useless substance. Over the years, men, women, and children who practice Natural Hygiene have stopped using it, and they're all better off for it. Furthermore, salt is a laxative because the body rejects it in fecal matter. Salt is an irritant; you need only rub salt in a wound to feel its burn.

"In the last century, numerous Natural Hygiene practitioners have raised herds of horses, sheep, and cows without feeding them salt because they knew that wild animals don't need salt. This proves that domestic animals don't need salt either.

"Personally," adds Shelton, "I have cows, horses, and other animals, and I have never given them salt. The results have been entirely satisfactory.

"I also raised my children without salt with excellent results."

In fact, Shelton was a farmer's son and had lots of animals.

Poisons in Moderation Too?

In the report which came to us from Moscow, it's worth noting that they only speak of the dangers of excessive salt consumption, but what exactly is excess? People who use salt following their sense of taste don't believe that they're using excessive amounts.

It's reminiscent of an adage which says, "Moderation in all things." Unfortunately, this maxim doesn't distinguish between healthy and unhealthy substances. Eating healthy food in moderation is probably fine, but should we take drugs in moderation? Tobacco? Coffee? Should we also lie in moderation?

Moderation is only acceptable for the healthy things in life. As for life's unhealthy aspects, moderation is unacceptable.

This is why eating salt, pepper and chemical products in moderation, as well as taking medication, is not a legitimate form of moderation.

"It's the same old mistake," says Shelton, "which would have us believe that poisons are only toxic once a certain amount – that is to say, they are just quantitatively dangerous, not qualitatively – rather than recognizing they are fundamentally and intrinsically dangerous.

"This way of thinking implies that salt, in moderation, is beneficial. Tribes of people, such as Native Americans, and even entire nations have lived for centuries without eating salt."

The Eskimo never had salt until the white man introduced the toxic substance to them.

Sunburn

Under the blazing sun of the Sahara, workers in oil wells must take salt tablets to prevent fatal heat strokes and less severe complications. This is easy to understand. Salt holds water within the body which protects it from excess heat.

These are exceptional conditions, and it is, of course, better to take these salt tablets than to die under the intense sun. In this case, it is a lesser evil.

I had an Italian friend in Cairo. During the summer, he played volleyball under the sun all day long wearing only a simple bathing suit. He was continually moving, but the sun did not leave him alone, and he came down with a high fever which lasted for several days and even threatened to take his life. It was a miracle that he survived. With salt tablets, he might have been able to avoid this heat stroke or at the very least reduced its severity. It's better to simply avoid both salt and intense sunlight.

Healthy bodies will react violently against poisonous substances, whereas a sick and intoxicated body will respond slowly. In the first case (that of the healthy body), the body's reaction can be so violent that death may follow. This won't be the case for the other person.

Salt Was Once Worth Gold?

In the past, people valued salt as highly as gold and silver. The same was true for spices which were even more unhealthy than salt. Does this indicate that these substances are useful, beneficial and vital for our bodies?

Human beings always suffer from sweet delusions. The greatest of these illusions is that of stimulants. We imagine that stimulants give us strength, but the opposite is true; they subtract from our power. Stimulation is deceitful. It is the same as whipping a tired horse; it seems to give the horse more energy as it runs faster, but it is exhausting the horse's strength, and it will thus collapse even sooner.

Organic Salt

Our bodies need salt, but it's an organic, plant—based and living salt. We find it in fruits and vegetables.

The way that vegetables are typically cooked (in a lot of water people throw out afterward) strip them of the minerals they contain, thus rendering the vegetables insipid. To maintain the natural salts contained in vegetables, they must be cooked in a minimal amount of water (only two or three cups of water) so that there is almost no water left at the end. In preparing them this way, you will find that vegetables have a naturally salty taste and you won't need to add table salt to them. They should also be cooked as little as possible because cooking transforms the living, plant—based organic minerals into inert, chemical, and unusable mineral salts.

The Taste of Food

Human beings, like other animals, recognize a food's value based on its salt and sugar content. Natural foods which are rich in minerals (salt) and sugar are superior to other natural foods which contain a meager amount of these substances. Highly sweet fruits are more valuable than bland fruits. We refuse to eat insipid melons. Some golden apples are simultaneously sugary and savory and are therefore among the most expensive. Certain varieties of tomatoes are naturally "saltier," whereas others are blander. Organic apples are "saltier" than those which come from forced production and are often insipid.

Unfortunately, our sense of taste is depraved and perverted due to tobacco, coffee, and a lousy diet. We can't differentiate between natural and industrial sugar any more than we can distinguish the natural salt contained in Swiss chard from table salt.

Instinctotherapy bases its health system on the notion of pure and natural instincts, didn't anticipate that the instincts of the overwhelming majority of people have become perverted.

> *__Note from the publisher:__ "Instinctive Eating" or in French "Instinctotherapy" was a popular raw food diet philosophy created by Guy—Claude Burger (pronounced Bur—Jher, with a soft "j," not like the English word "burger"), but had a very small impact in the United States, where only a few books on the topic were published and one community/retreat center was formed on the Big Island of Hawaii. The idea was to only eat raw foods, eat them one at a time until full, and select them by smell. In this system, everything raw was allowed: fruits, vegetables, honey, nuts, raw meat, oysters, and even raw chicken! The movement more or less ended when Burger was thrown in jail after a big pedophilia scandal that shocked France. When Mosséri wrote his books, Instinctotherapy was still very popular, although many of its followers suffered health problems as a result.*

For those who do have pure instincts, the taste of artificial sugar hurts the throat as it is violent. The same is true for salt. Natural and healthy foods never have a strong taste.

Even animals, whose instincts are purer than our own, are enticed and fooled by the taste of industrial sugar and table salt. It seems that they go to lick salt flats. In short, without plant—based sugar and salt, humans beings cannot survive.

Salt Advocates

Naturopaths have always allowed for Celtic or other types of sea salt when consumed in moderation. Some people talk about salt *vitalization* by natural elements. How is it vitalized? They don't say. Is sea salt transformed into organic salt with the help of natural elements, and if so, which ones?

Practitioner A. Passebecq refutes this argument by saying, "As for the vitalization process of sea salt and mineral substances which occur in the earth and ocean water, our stance remains doubtful… are these substances absorbed by our cells? Inorganic substances can't be assimilated unless they come from a plant." We understand the term "inorganic" to mean chemical.

This is the principal argument against salt. Salt is a chemical, mineral substance that the body cannot assimilate unless it comes from a plant, which transforms it into an organic element. Humans do not have this ability. Only plants can do this. Only plants can digest mineral salts and offer them to us in an organic, plant—based and living form. Cooking salt is an inert, chemical product that, no different from other chemical products.

> **Notes from the publisher:** The statement that table or sea salt is not assimilated because it's not "organic," or doesn't come from a plant, is inaccurate, but was an early theory originating in the early writings of Natural Hygienists. In reality the problem with salt is that it is assimilated, and this causes a great sodium imbalance in the body. So the only thing Natural Hygiene got wrong was the operating principle. They were perfectly aware of the consequences.

Let's look at other arguments raised by one of the most prestigious naturopaths at the turn of the century, Dr. Paul Carton.

One of Dr. Carton's mistakes, among many others, unfortunately, advocated salt. Dr. Carton was a genuine researcher, but he was too full of himself and plagiarized Mono (**NFP**: another nutritionist of the past) behind closed doors while ignoring work of Natural Hygiene researchers because they were "foreign." He thought of himself as the center of the universe.

Being a tuberculosis patient, he was opposed to fasting. But not everyone in the world has tuberculosis.

"The need for salt which airborne animals feel more, or less urgently," he writes," is an automatic ancestral reminder, and therefore, it's legitimate. Mammals are especially quite fond of salt. Poultry farmers noticed that using salt in moderation in their chicken feed was most useful for appetite stimulation and caused the food to be better assimilated."

It's true that from time to time, animals lick salt and even seek it out. However, this is in no way proof that this practice is legitimate, and it doesn't demonstrate a physiological need. In fact, animals, like humans, are fooled by these substances, and while their instinct is less perverted than ours, that doesn't mean it's immune to making mistakes. Animals often commit mistakes in their diets; just like humans, they are attracted and fooled by the stimulation provoked by salt and white sugar. They can't distinguish plant—based salt from chemical salt and natural sugar from industrial sugar.

Moreover, if poultry farmers put salt in their chicken feed and then noticed that their chickens ate more, it's because they had no control over what they were eating. The salted food rapidly passes through their body as droppings while their intestines simultaneously reject the food bolus. As a result, the food the food provides no benefit to the poultry, and they eat even more. Furthermore, if the chicken is then fatter and thus more profitable, it's because all the salt causes water retention. Tissues drenched in water and salt are unhealthy.

"It seems," Carton continues, "that some monasteries were able to eliminate all harmful stimulants; at the same time, they were never able to eliminate salt."

Is there such a thing as harmful vs. healthy stimulants? All stimulants are harmful! It's essential to understand that in this example from Dr. Carton, wine and beer were allowed in monasteries, but he considered that these were good stimulants. Natural Hygiene practitioners reject wine and beer as being unhealthy alcoholic beverages.

Furthermore, we can't consider the diet served in even the most austere monasteries as being healthy. Multitudes of Natural Hygiene practitioners have given up salt long ago, and they haven't experienced any negative consequences as a result. They drank neither wine nor beer! Moreover, when we eat fruits and raw vegetables, we do not need salt.

Wasn't it Dr. Carton who advised cooking vegetables in several successive pots of water to draw out all the "excessive" natural minerals they contained? What ignorance! Natural foods don't include anything in excess. They are perfect as they are.

After having changed the cooking water three times, Carton advised replacing the natural minerals (lost in cooking) with table salt! It goes without saying that vegetables which have been cooked in this way no longer have any taste.

It's a mistake to believe that natural foods contain too much sodium, implying that they damage the body. However, even if we assume that Dr. Carton is correct and vegetables are too concentrated, we would only need to eat three times less! That would be more logical than stripping them of their natural, plant—based, organic and living salts to replace them with a dead, chemical and mineral salt.

Salt Vitalization

"Sodium chloride, a vital and universal salt built by life itself, remains undecomposed across both land—based and aquatic environments where it is vitalized by microbial processes and rendered digestible, just like other mineral products…;"

This point of view is more romantic than scientific. It isn't right that microbial processes *vitalize* chemical salt, nor is it true that these salts are digestible for human beings. In fact, the body rejects the salt through sweat, urine, and tears.

Dr. Carton was fooling himself with his vague notions of vitalization. This same reasoning could justify consuming so many other inert minerals, such as volcanic lava, limestone, and pulverized rocks!

On the contrary, living foods must decompose, and if salt reminds undecomposed (in Dr. Carton's terms), that is a sign that it is neither living nor vitalized. The ideas of the old doctor on this subject were quite confusing.

This reminds me of some naturopaths in India with whom I stayed in 1949 to study naturopathy. I don't know if this habit is unique to India or only to Indian naturopaths, but they had the habit of only drinking fresh water – that is, water drawn from the well just before drinking it. According to them, water that had been pulled from the well the day before must not be consumed because it was no longer fresh and had lost its vitality. Even in France, in some circles, people sell "vitalized" water. It's a fraud. It also extends to the reasoning that homeopaths use to justify their useless practices.

Magnesium chloride is undoubtedly not an organic, vital salt like Dr. Carton says (short of finding it in food, of course). Dr. Carton is talking about table salt. This salt is chemical, dead and inert. Plants vitalize it when they absorb it and transform it.

However, even plants can only absorb small quantities of it. When drenched in salted water, plants die.

Sodium chloride is not built by life itself as Dr. Carton pretends it to be. In fact, chemical transformations have nothing to do with life. What about coal? Didn't life create it? It comes from wood which was once a living plant but is no longer. Should we eat that as well?

Contrary to what Dr. Carton says, table salt hasn't undergone any "stage" of microbial vitalization, just like coal and chalk. If it has, I'd like to know which one.

Sodium chloride (salt) is a considerable interference in "bodily exchanges and secretions." In fact, it forces the body to retain more liquid than it would otherwise need which overwhelms it and hinders its processes. The presence of table salt within the body presents a considerable obstacle for bodily exchanges because it is a foreign substance. According to Pavlov, even secretions are inhibited and the composition of saliva changes. Saliva becomes primarily composed of water to dilute salts which would otherwise irritate. It ceases to contain enzymes; it is no longer active saliva but an imitation.

Finally, Dr. Carton claims that "salt is digestible, just like other minerals," but chemical minerals are not digestible at all; they are rejected.

Stimulation Through Salt

Table salt, being neither digestible nor capable of being assimilated, must be eliminated from our body. The kidneys are responsible for disposing of retained water. This additional work exhausts them, often to the point of renal degeneration and lesions.

People say that salt is an "energy producer and activates nutrient metabolism." This is a significant error. This is false stimulation which we only imagine provides us with energy. What a beautiful delusion! When you're tired, and you drink a cup of coffee, you immediately feel your energy come back. When you are still half—awake, coffee wakes you up and gets you on your feet. Would you say that coffee produces energy?

An exhausted horse will run quicker when whipping it, but does the energy come from the whip? No.

Poisons, stimulants, coffee, salt, and whips all cause the body to expend more of its stored energy thus taking that energy away from poison elimination processes. This constitutes a loss of energy which, in the end, causes the body to collapse even faster.

The energy that the body expends to rid itself of the poisons we call stimulants is not an energy gain but an expenditure of energy reserves.

Coffee and salt do not give energy; on the contrary, they take away and squander our energy. The activity observed following their consumption comes from the body's effort to eliminate them. It's an exhausting activity.

Selective Osmosis

Cooking salt doesn't help with "osmotic exchanges." Furthermore, is there a type of osmosis which occurs within the body as we observe it in laboratories? Certainly not.

The type of osmosis which occurs within the body is more of a selective "osmosis" which is neither blind nor chemical. Even this osmosis is hindered by the presence of foreign matter within the body.

The intestines absorb nutritive matter, but they resist useless substances.

"It is only when salt is nothing more than a practically inert chemical body, having lost all potential vitalization energy that it had acquired in land—based and aquatic environments, that it is eliminated."

This is pure romanticism. Dr. Carton finally recognized that salt is, in the end, eliminated, indicating that it serves no purpose.

As for the "potential vitalization energy" in question, this is a rather vague and confusing notion which certainly comes from the spiritual world. It hasn't been proven that chemical products, including salt, can be "vitalized." In this realm, spiritual interrogations only serve to create confusion within the mind.

On the other hand, when a plant digests an inert salt, the plant transforms it into a plant—based salt; it vitalizes it and renders it organic.

Antibiotic Salt

Of course, salt is an antibiotic. In brines, vegetables die within a few days because salt kills life. Antibiotic means "against life." "Bio" comes from the Latin word meaning life.

Antibiotics kill precious bacteria in the intestinal flora, and salt also has this effect.

The Symptoms Which Follow the Elimination of Salt

"Eliminating salt from a human's diet," said Dr. Carton, "is immediately followed by problems: fatigue, loss of appetite, digestive difficulties due to a depletion of gastric juices, weakening of the immune system, seeking compensatory stimulants to attain the same physiological response we get from salt..."

Let's look at all of these problems Dr. Carton mentions one—by—one as some of them are delusions while others are merely poor interpretation:

Fatigue

In fact, it is likely that eliminating salt will lead to a certain level of fatigue. Is this a problem? The immediate suppression of any stimulant will cause the body to lower the amount of energy it would ordinarily employ to get rid of the stimulant. This fatigue – instead, this *relaxation* – is therefore beneficial in and of itself. It signifies the end of the body's useless squandering of strength and its gradual recuperation. This fatigue disappears after a few weeks of perseverance; therefore, it is temporary. The solution is to rest.

A person will feel a similar sense of fatigue – *relaxation* – when eliminating bread and meat from the diet. This fatigue – *relaxation* – can last for several months. It's important not to become discouraged but to persevere.

Not only will the energy wholly and forcefully return, but the weight will also go back to normal. The solution is to rest further and not shake it off. This allows the body to adapt quicker.

Dr. Carton didn't look far enough because the immediate effects are somewhat deceptive. In fact, "the law of duality" cited in my book, *Entrust Your Health to Nature*, stipulates:

"Every foreign substance introduced into the body will, over time, occasion double and contrary reaction: the reaction will be the opposite of the first action."

This is why tonics "strengthen" but later weaken the body. Alcohol "stimulates," only to later depress. Everything which temporarily strengthens the body will weaken it in the long term."

I eliminated salt from diet 40 years ago, and I've had no problems. Nevertheless, I have been tempted by a multitude of sugary and salty products sold in supermarkets. To avoid these tantalizing products, I had powdered vegetable soup after dinner for many months. It was the salt that attracted me by giving me that pleasant stimulation.

After a few months, I began to feel tingling in my feet which worried me day and night.

It woke me up every night. I even had an automobile accident because of the tingling as I was unable to drive my car and scratch myself at the same time. Mustard and spices always immediately made my hair stand on end from the tingling in my scalp.

Thus, I attributed these trouble to salt as well as to the MSG that was probably in the soup. I had to abstain from salt for four weeks for these unpleasant problems to disappear.

It seems that in health food stores, it's possible to find vegetable soups without salt or MSG.

Thus, it would be interesting to instantly prepare these soups in the morning as a coffee replacement.

Loss of Appetite

Salt advocates say that eliminating salt from your leads to a loss of appetite. What does that mean? It means that you weren't truly hungry!

Moreover, with our taste largely blunted, how are we supposed to taste foods in their natural state? When we smoke, we are no longer able to taste anything. Fast and your appetite will return after a few days.

When we salty foods, we are tempted to scarf down twice as much to remedy the irritation that the salt causes.

Digestive Difficulties

Dr. Carton suggests that eliminating salt leads to digestive difficulties. Is this true?

In fact, we do observe some difficulties, but we must instead view them as a good thing. In reality, the body is making an effort to digest the food after eliminating salt. We sometimes feel heaviness and malaise as a result, but this is temporary.

With salt, on the other hand, food is rapidly directed to the colon with almost no digestion because the body is pressed to get rid of the salt. The body only digests a part of the food; the individual feels nothing; they are content. The person will say that they had no digestive difficulties, but in reality, they didn't digest much. This is why he doesn't feel any difficulties!

When you eliminate salt, your body will improve its digestion. Each week, it will digest more than the week before, and because of it, you will no longer need lots of food and will suffer less.

Conclusive experiments proved that salt delays digestion and prevents the production of digestive diastase (enzymes).

This indicates to us that the quantity of food which is not digested, eaten with salt, will end up irritating our intestinal lining and poisoning our body. The inevitable putrefaction and fermentation which occurs provoke illnesses resulting from toxemia.

In the same manner of thinking, we often advise taking a walk before going to bed to avoid digestive difficulties. This advice is understandable because during the night, energy begins to slow and digestion could become stalled.

Once again, let us repeat that heaviness is the body attempting to digest food.

Weakened Immune System

Dr. Carton suggests that eliminating salt leads to a weakened immune system.

The term "weakened immune system" denotes medical obscurantism which considers illness as an external attack. Modern medicine doesn't understand the elimination purpose of illness. It's like talking to a brick wall.

For those who have eliminated stimulants from their diet, detoxification crises are beneficial and useful events. Modern medicine will never understand that and will always seek to reduce symptoms in which they see only as bad.

If, after you eliminate all stimulants from your diet — salt, coffee, spices, wine — and modify your way of eating, you come down with a high fever, a doctor will tell you that you have developed a weakened immune system. This strikes fear into people who then submit to antibiotics without even flinching.

These detoxification crises are always beneficial, even when they take the form of an illness which is well—known within the medical community. Don't let them fool you. Medicine is not a science. All of its notions are false. Let's not forget that Dr. Carton was a medical doctor – that is, he was handicapped by his medical training.

The term "weakened immune system" clearly emphasizes the erroneous medical notion that illness comes from the world around us, from a microbial attack. However, our Natural Hygiene conception is opposed to this notion. Microbes are not the cause, even in a favorable environment. Internal toxemia is the cause – that is to say, the environment. – "Microbes are nothing; the terrain is everything."

Seeking Compensatory Stimulants to Get the Same Physiological Response That We Get From Salt

A person has liver disease. You have them eliminate wine from their diet, and they switch to beer. This isn't serious.

When someone eliminates a stimulant like salt from their diet, they must wait to feel the withdrawal effects of the irritant – that is a certain degree of fatigue. With a bit of perseverance, the body adapts, and the fatigue disappears. We mustn't replace one poison with another. We must eliminate all stimulants: coffee, wine, pepper, mustard, etc.

We absolutely must not seek something else to stimulate ourselves. We must accept the temporary fatigue and rest.

Speaking of the "physiological" action of salt, this implies that an inert substance act on the body. According to Thrall's Law, outlined in my book *Entrust Your Health to Nature*
"Each time an action is carried out within a living organism as the result of an exterior influence, the action must be attributed to the living thing which has the power to act, not the inert, inanimate thing whose principal characteristic is its inertia."

Thus, we see that salt doesn't act on the body, but instead, the latter acts upon the former to eliminate it. Even food has no action on the body; it is the latter which acts upon them to digest, absorb and assimilate them.

Therefore, it would be correct to say that salt has a pathological effect.

CHAPTER 2: No Bread, No Grains

All real natural hygiene practitioners are against grains, including bread, rice, pasta, starches, cookies, etc. However, I spent a decade trying to understand the reasons to be able to put this dietary rule into practice. It is challenging to understand this subject because, unconsciously, we refuse to abandon our habit of eating bread and grains.

Nutritionists who accept bread, even whole—grain, are not real advocates of Natural Hygiene. On the other hand, I receive numerous letters from readers saying that they do not understand why I would be against whole—grain bread.

They don't understand that nature does not produce bread and that grains are meant to be eaten by granivorous birds while human beings are frugivorous.

It was in 1950 when I was 25 years old that I made several prolonged and unsuccessful attempts to eliminate bread from my diet. To compensate, I threw myself at all types of cookies and cakes. I followed the bad advice that I shouldn't eat between meals, in spite of my hunger.

My understanding was incomplete, and my diet was chaotic. In fact, chronic partial indigestion causes a pressing desire to eat which, in time, is followed by meals which are too consistent and provoke another bout of heartburn in a vicious, never—ending circle.

There are many reasons not to eat grains, but in my opinion, those which are most valuable are those which are based in biology – that is to say, those arguments which are invoked by vegetarians when speaking out against meat.

In fact, the Table of *Comparative Anatomy and Physiology*, which we will study in my next book, emphasizes that human beings do not have the characteristics of carnivores. They do not have the canine teeth necessary to crush flesh, the claws required to tear it apart, a stomach which is powerful enough to digest meat, nor a large enough liver to neutralize the toxins meats contain, and so forth.

This is something that everyone can easily understand: human beings are not carnivorous. However, when I emphasize that human beings also lack the characteristics of granivorous animals, people begin to raise their hands as they no longer understand what I'm saying.

For each class of animals on Earth, Nature anticipated a particular category of foods perfectly adapted for them, and any derogation from this order will lead to physiological disturbances – illnesses, degeneration, cancer.

A machine which is meant to function with a particular kind of oil will not function as well with a different type of oil. It will clog the machine and wear it out.

This is the fundamental argument which we must keep in mind against grains. All other so—called scientific arguments are only details.

Nature foresaw that fish would have a special kind of diet, reptiles would have their own, cows would have a third fare, lions would have a carnivorous diet and primates also their particular diet.

Nature is no chaos. Each species of animal eats the food which Nature intended for it to eat, and they do not infringe upon the food of other species. If a horse were to begin to eat meat and a lion were to eat grass, that would be the end of everything.

For example, we currently feed chickens a carnivorous diet. In fact, the industrial powders we feet them contain animal waste, coming from slaughterhouses. This causes their eggs to contain dangerous bacteria: salmonella.

Human Beings Are Fruitarian

"It's interesting to remember," Mr. Clements writes in the June 1971 issue of the journal *Health for All* (London), "that toward the end of the last century, our country had a *Natural Food Society* whose purpose was as follows:

"The Natural Food Society is founded on the conviction that humanity's original food consisted of fruit and nuts which grew in temperate regions; it was on these foods that human beings existed, free from the illnesses that no animal experiences in their natural state.

"The Society's principal belief was that grains are not natural for human consumption and lead to illness. This is the primary cause of the anxiety, fatigue and health degeneration that we see all around us…"

This diet was founded by the famous Dr. Emmet Densmore and his wife, Hélène. It advocated for a grain—free diet of fruit. However, Dr. Densmore found that in England, there wasn't enough fruit for people to be able to sustain themselves year—round. That was 100 years ago, but things have changed a great deal since that time. Now, we can find oranges and grapefruits year—round. Currently, global transportation is rapid and brings fruit to all corners of the earth.

In France, we have mangoes, kiwis, avocados, grapes, peaches, apples, and pears practically year—round.

Of course, fruit is more expensive than bread, and grapes are more expensive than wine!

It's a paradox of our capitalist civilization that these end products are more expensive than the primary material from which they were made.

According to Dr. Kellogg John Harvey, fruit and various nuts constitute an ideal diet to support human life for its average span. We should specify that the average human lifespan is at least 120 years.

Nevertheless, in 1964, Dr. George Schaller discovered that gorillas do not eat various nuts and bananas.

This suggests that these foods are not as useful for gorillas as they are for other kinds of monkeys, and therefore, they are not as useful for human beings. Consuming these foods (nuts) in excess leads to gas and putrefaction.

"Fruits," writes Dr. Vetrano, "are a precious source of energy which surpasses even starches because they require less energy to digest. In fact, scientific experiments have shown for a long time that fructose is the most economical source of body heat and energy.

"On the other hand, refined white sugar, or high—fructose corn syrup steal alkaline elements from the body, whereas in fruit, their natural, organic sugars and acids are combined with enough alkaline mineral salts to neutralize the acidity formed during metabolism."

In 1923, Otto Carque wrote *Rational Diet*, in which he compared white sugar with fruit sugar:

"Although their composition is identical, fruit sugar is intimately associated with essential elements which are crucial for neutralizing the acid that arises from its oxidation in the body, whereas refined sugar, although it can temporarily act as a stimulant, cannot maintain the body's vital processes.

"In fact, when we ingest refined, industrial sugar, our body's cells are rapidly disintegrated to give the blood the alkaline elements it needs to clear the acids which result from its combustion. This explains why a body nourished with devitalized foods will break down quicker than if it had been subjected to an absolute fast.

"Natural Hygiene practitioners," Dr. Vetrano continues, "prefer fruit as a source of carbohydrates rather than grains, not only because is is simple to digest but also because of its superior nutritive value."

In fact, grains and bread, even whole—grain bread, are quite deficient in mineral salts and alkaline minerals, such as calcium, when compared to fruit. In fact, their digestion steals calcium from the body. Therefore, they are decalcifying, in particular, because of the phytic acid they contain. They combine with the calcium contained in food, rendering it insoluble and indigestible.

Moreover, the sugar contained in fruit is easy to digest. It is predigested, whereas starches require a long time to process to be transformed into glucose. This glucose enters the blood too quickly which explains the "slump" we feel after eating bread, followed by stimulation – thus, many highs and lows.

Fruit is always alkalizing when is is digested well, whereas bread, even whole—grain bread, and grains are always acidifying.

In fact, metabolic waste coming from fruit contains sodium, potassium, calcium and magnesium salts, whereas waste from digested bread primarily contains sulfur, chloride, and phosphorus which are all acidifying.

Obese people can lose weight by replacing grains with fruit. On the other hand, thin people can gain weight by eliminating grains and replacing them with fruit. In fact, those who have a healthy digestive system can gain weight with grains, while those who have a weak digestive system would be quickly overwhelmed and exhausted by the problematic digestion associated with starches and would thus maintain their thin weight.

In conclusion, with fruit, we can maintain an ideal weight whereas, with grains, a person will either gain or lose weight by the strength of their digestive system.

We can easily see this by monitoring the weight of a fasting person when they begin to eat again. Without including starches in the diet, we notice that the person who has fasted will regularly gain weight until it reaches the healthy weight.

Finally, fruit can be eaten raw, whereas it is tough to eat raw grains. We know that cooking destroys vitamins and mineral salts, in bread and grains – they already contain very little of these substances.

No animal, except for human beings, eats cooked foods. Cooking is not natural. Birds find raw grains pleasant to see and to eat, whereas human beings cannot savor them without sugaring, salting and cooking which denatures them.

CHAPTER 3: Did Humans Adapt to Eat Meat and Bread?

In a future chapter, we will study comparative anatomy and physiology according to famous works by famous anatomists, including Sir Charles Bell, Dr. Richard Owen, Dr. William Carpenter and Baron Cuvier.

From this research, it is evident that we should classify human beings as vegetarians – that is, they should be living off fruit, vegetables, and greens.

In short, carnivores possess a dental composition which allows them to kill their prey with their very long and razor—sharp canine teeth; their intestines are shorter than those of herbivores, and as a result, they cannot graze on grass. Their intestines would need to be much longer to process it. Their stomach and liver are both enormous and powerful, and therefore, they can neutralize all of the toxins in meat. Moreover, in addition to many other fascinating details, carnivores eat raw meat.

Human beings, on the other hand, are designed to feed off fruits and vegetables, just like certain machines can only function with certain kinds of fuels. The human anatomical structure has adapted to a diet of fruits, vegetables, and greens.

Adaptation

People will reply that humans have finally adapted to a meat—based diet, after having eaten meat for thousands of years.

In reality, humanity has yet to see its hair grow out to the point of becoming bushy; we are still not covered with furs like lions and tigers. We also still lack canines long enough and sharp enough to be considered beasts of prey. The length of our intestines has yet to change or evolve. It is the same as it has been for all these centuries. We have yet to obtain claws for killing and tearing the flesh of our prey.

In short, there has been no such evolution.

Changes Which Have Arisen

Of course, there have been some changes to the human body after such a diet of meat and bread, but we cannot call these changes evolution because they are nothing more than pathological changes.

What exactly are the changes that take place when a person follows a diet of bread and meat? To put it simply, they're chronic illnesses and all the consequences associated with them!

This is how the body tolerates and evolve to tobacco and meat, but we can't say that the body has to evolve to eating fruit.

We need only look at one example: people who have developed a tolerance for and adapted to arsenic to the point that their body can absorb doses that would kill most people. The same is true for tobacco, meat, and bread. A person who is smoking for the first time is incapable of going through several packs a day like chain—smokers often do.

This type of evolution or adaptation occurs via changes in the tissue which only leads the body further from what is ideal (i.e., it leads to lung cancer, stomach ulcers, etc.). It's not advantageous to be able to withstand doses of poison which would kill the average person. Those who have adapted to these toxic substances are more dead than alive.

In the past, people rarely ate meat – that is, it was consumed at most once a week or once a month. In Egypt, peasants, who made up the majority of the population, only ate meat twice each year during festivals and after the Ramadan (the one—month muslim fast).

However, in this affluent day and age, people in Europe eat meat every day, sometimes multiple times per day. I knew a Canadian who ate several different types of meat (ham, beef, chicken, fish, etc.) as often as five times per day. This diet was coupled with frequent antibiotic usage, and in the end, he developed severe health problems. He had to stop taking antibiotics, stop eating meat and undergo a curative fast to fully recover.

Nowadays, we have entire generations of people who have regularly and frequently eaten meat for centuries, but as a result of this, we also see cancer, which is a direct consequence of this diet.

Degeneration and cancer: these are Nature's means of adaptation.

These are the ultimate consequences of such a diet, but of course, there is an entire range of intermediary medical conditions, such as sinusitis, asthma, hepatitis, ulcers, mental illnesses, etc. These conditions occur over the course of several years spent groaning and suffering. We mustn't waste these years in silence like the famous people whose deaths we read about in the media. We don't address all the years of suffering that the deceased had to endure, choosing instead to rapidly mention the vague name of their illness, followed by the announcement of their death.

Three Kinds of Adaptation

Shelton once said that the word adaptation is a magic word that conceals ignorance and bias. He mercilessly refuted this so—called argument which has no scientific value. Let's look at what he said on this subject, for his writings are invaluable. Vegetarian movements would be better off turning to these books for inspiration, rather than standing by their weak, superficial arguments.

"The term adaptation has a very vague meaning and commonly used in a variety of ways. Depending on how we use the word, it can express ideas that are as disparate as the opinions of those representing them!

1) Here are some examples of the first kind of adaptation:

- Muscle enlargement following exercise
- Skin becoming tan when exposed to the sun
- Hardening of skin on the palms of the hands and soles of the feet when following hard labor

2) Here are examples of the second kind of adaptation:
- Wearing more clothes when it's cold outside
- Seeking shelter when it is raining or when there is thunder

3) Finally, here are some examples of the third kind of adaptation which we will refer to as tolerance:
- The acquired ability to smoke without suffering from any acute symptoms and to ingest enough arsenic to kill several people without immediate dying." – Shelton

Exaggeration or Decline

Admittedly, we know very little about the body's "adaptation mechanism," but it's clear that most of these adaptations are merely the exaggeration or decline of standard structures and functions.

Examples of this include our skin tanning when exposed to the sun and our muscles growing after exercise. Some animals have fur which protects them from harsh winters. This is a well—known example of a structural exaggeration which has resulted in an adaptation process.

Is the Adaptation Useful Or Harmful?

We commonly say that human beings are adaptable and subject to considerable change, but we shouldn't deduce from this that each of these adaptations is necessarily beneficial and useful, nor should we assume that it is in our best interest.

A Double-Edged Sword

Adaptation is like a double-edged sword. For example, it can ensure that we have some protection against poisons such as tobacco, arsenic, or alcohol, but at the same time, it can reduce our functional abilities and harm their associated structures. In fact, adaptations are always accomplished through changes which lead the body away from its ideal state. As a result, the thickening and hardening of protective membranes also reduce the functional capacity of the affected tissues.

For example, the lungs can adapt to tobacco use, but this leads them to develop cancer – a fact that is well-known by smokers – as well as heart disease, amblyopia, etc. Tobacco alters our sense of taste and smell; we are less capable of savoring our foods. It's clear that this type of pathological adaptation is only an illusion.

Until tobacco use becomes a habit, it's disgusting and not even remotely attractive. The same is true for other poisons: tea, coffee, alcohol, cocoa, chocolate and betel (used in India). They are all repulsive to those whose sense of taste has not become depraved.

These people also find fermented beer terrible. Wine is disgusting to them. Should they acquire a taste for these horrible beverages? I have never liked wine, champagne, beer, and coffee.

Human Beings Don't Have to Adapt to Eat Healthy Foods!

"Human beings don't need to adapt to the healthy aspects of their lives. Furthermore, they don't have to acquire a taste for natural foods, water, and pure air.

"These things can be used without causing any changes to the tissue which would cause the body to stray from its ideal state. When used legitimately, they will not change vital structures or functions. They are pleasant to people with a normal sense of taste and smell. These people do not have to undergo any undesirable pathological changes to enjoy these foods." – Shelton.

"Human beings don't need to adapt to the healthy aspects of their lives," writes Shelton in this brilliant paper. Furthermore, people who replace alcohol with water, polluted city air with the pure air of the country and artificial foods with natural options should see their body adapt through changes which bring it closer to its normal, ideal state of health.

Alas, when pathological changes have become too advanced, and the associated illnesses have also become chronic, so long as no irreversible conditions have arisen, the road to recovery will be long.

Though the journey will be long, it won't be impossible. It only requires persistence and perseverance. The patient must be determined to restore their health, regardless of what obstacles they may face.

Wonderful Cultural Adaptations

"It is said," says Shelton in his analysis, "that human beings were particularly gifted at making changes to the world around them when they colonized the earth. In fact, this colonization was made possible not by changes within the human body but by modifications enacted in their environment. Human beings seem to be more capable of adapting nature to suit their needs than of adapting themselves to suit nature. Thus, humans created clothing, built houses, learned to make fire, invented air conditioning and began to do many other things to live comfortably, regardless of the climate in which they lived.

"The most useful and healthy adaptations were more cultural than biological. Rather than growing thick fur on their skin when moving to colder regions, humans learned to build homes, wear clothes and warm themselves up. With no fur covering their bodies, rather than becoming hairy creatures, humans became weavers and tailors! Rather than storing fat for hibernation or becoming a seasonally migratory species, humanity learned how to save food for the winter. Human beings lack the fangs and claws that are necessary to trap and kill prey, but to compensate; they have learned how to create tools and weapons.

"Since human beings don't have snouts, like pigs, with which they can move earth, they invented tools with which they can dig. They cultivated the earth to increase their production abilities. They learned to irrigate, to dig deeply into the earth in search of water and to transport food and water across long distances.

"They domesticated many different animals. When migrating, they transported animals and plants which served their needs.

"In short, humanity changed its environment rather than itself. The ability to transform one's environment – which many other animals possess to a lesser degree – has been the biggest asset for survival. Biological adaptation, on the other hand, had played a minor role in human life. Rather than undergoing physiological changes to adapt to various environments, humans have merely adapted their environment to themselves. Humans can live in both tropical and glacial climates not because their bodies have adapted but because they have been able to create a cultural environment in which they can survive.

"Gorillas are very strong, but they are incapable of adapting to the various climates and physical conditions in which humanity has learned to survive. This is because they have not undergone the biological adaptation or another form of adaptation (i.e., cultural adaptation) that this would require. They are very limited in where they can live. Human beings are supreme beings because they can adapt culturally.

"Humans have managed to survive in unfavorable and difficult situations, but it has always been at the expense of their strength, endurance, and longevity." – Dr. H.M. Shelton.

Ecology

"We now arrive at civilized humanity. Why must we ask modern humans to adapt to the evils that exist in our civilization? Instead, why not make humanity the center of our universe and adapt our civilization to human needs?"

Ecologists have understood this, and as a result, they fight against nuclear power plants and electrical, atmospheric and chemical pollution. They aren't interested in food pollution – at least, not yet.

"Humanity's cultural acquisitions have not been favorable to its well—being. In fact, a large part of what we refer to as progress and civilization is definitively opposed to health, vigor, strength, mental equilibrium, and longevity. Examples of these include industrial manufacturing, chemical pollution of natural foods, many toxic habits, medical practices, most surgical operations, staying up late and many other habits which are destructive to our health." – Hygienic Review, Vol. 32, No. 10.

Humans Are Not Adapted to Carnivorous and Grain-Based Diets

"The biological principle that a particular anatomical structure will correlate with a particular way of obtaining food and with a kind of food seems to be to be in perfect harmony with a multitude of other biological facts, such as we know them today.

"If we look at human beings strictly as animals or zoological specimens, we are forced, by all the facts of comparative anatomy and physiology, to classify them as frugivorous." – Dr. H.M. Shelton.

CHAPTER 4: Can We Enjoy Meat?

Dr. Sh elton made the following proposition:

"Considering humanity's taste for fruit as normal and appropriate while considering the taste some humans have for meat as acquired certainly aligns better with the facts of comparative anatomy than the notion that human beings are carnivores who have adopted the habits of non—carnivorous species."

Shelton's statement also applies to grains, including bread.

We cannot say that humans enjoy eating grains, bread, pasta or rice in their natural state any more than we can say that humans enjoy eating meat and fish in their natural state.

When we eat meats, grains, and bread, we turn to seasonings, salt, sauces, cooking and other forms of processing just to make them edible.

Practically no one finds raw meat appetizing. Wheat grains are only appealing to birds.

"We must consider humanity's frugivorous tendencies as normal and appropriate while relegating their carnivorous practices as something acquired from a force of circumstances. We must push aside the idea that human beings are carnivores or omnivores."

We must also push aside the idea that human beings are granivores like birds are. In reality, humanity's frugivorous tendencies are healthy and appropriate, whereas its granivorous practices are a habit acquired from circumstances.

What exactly were these circumstances which forced the humans of yesteryear to eat meat and bread?

When war breaks out or drought dries up the earth, harvests practically non—existent. We cannot store fruit for long periods of time, but flour, on the other hand, can be kept for months. As a result, it can save entire populations from famine.

Nowadays, thanks to our technological progress, we can refrigerate apples and for a year or longer. This process could potentially be expanded to include other fruits, though not all of them.

It is preferable to even frozen fruit rather than meat, bread, and grains. In fact, the amount of vitamins in frozen fruits is far superior to that of meat, bread, and grains, which must be cooked at temperatures varying from 100o C to 250o C.

We are also able to dry out figs, dates, bananas, and grapes, and all of these dried fruits are superior to bread.

Adaptation = Deterioration

"The argument in favor of a carnivorous human diet due to the human body's ability to adapt is implicitly based on the notion that it's somehow desirable for human beings to take a step backward.

"It is a well—established fact that acquired characteristics cannot be genetically transmitted and inherited.

"Therefore, we must also accept that the functional adjustments necessary for humans to adapt to a meat—based diet are limited to each and cannot be transmitted genetically."

There are digestive differences between different individuals, but these differences aren't fundamental. At most, they are functional, and they do not justify completely different diets. As we have said, they are adjustments, not new functions.

These so—called adjustments are not physiological; instead, they are pathological changes which occur as soon as our diet strays from the ideal, Natural Hygienist diet for which humanity was designed.

On the other hand, when dietary changes are made to grow closer to the Natural Hygienist ideal, the changes which occur are physiological.

"It's important to understand that the changes we endure to adapt to a change in our condition do not always work in our favor.

"Favorable conditions tend to strengthen our body, whereas unfavorable conditions tend to exhaust and overwhelm it.

"Thus, several changes, referred to as adaptations, are likely to diminish the body's strength. If these unfavorable conditions continue, yielding proportional deterioration, disorganization and death will be waiting at the end of the road.

"Finally, if several generations were to be subjected to such unfavorable conditions, the extinction of the lineage could ultimately occur." Vol. 32, No. 10, Hygienic Review.

CHAPTER 5: Can We Develop a Tolerance to Wine, Coffee, and Anxiolytics?

According to Bastedo, an authority in pharmacology from the University of California, it seems that "wine, when consumed in moderate quantities, is absorbed in the stomach and intestines without ever reaching the colon. In those who drink wine regularly, this absorption is slowed." – Materia Medica, Pharmacology and Therapeutics.

"With that being said, Bastedo does not go on to explain how this alcohol absorption is slowed in those who drink wine regularly. It's clear that this delay is accomplished through changes which make the tissue impermeable to alcohol. Tissues suffer from induration which affects the gastrointestinal mucus lining the digestive tract.

This induration is the mechanism through which alcohol absorption is prevented.

"All pharmacologists would agree that alcohol is an irritant, and we know that induration (hardening) is the body's primary defense against chronic irritation.

"This defense is then mistaken for tolerance.

"Another form of additional and immediate protection which prevents alcohol absorption, even among those who do not drink it regularly, is reddening stomach mucus congestion followed by the secretion of a thick, sturdy and protective mucus. According to pharmacologists, this mucus not only protects the stomach lining against the destruction caused by alcohol, but it also slows absorption, thus protecting the liver and diminishing the harm to the body. It also sees as though drug users can eliminate alcohol from their body more quickly.

"When consumed in large quantities, alcohol leads to gastritis and alters digestion so greatly that it affects the appetite for several days after its ingestion. When consumed regularly, this gastritis becomes chronic. Chronic congestion and mucus secretion serve as constant obstacles to absorption. Moreover, chronic congestion cannot continue for long periods of time without causing harmful changes to the tissue.

"This goes back to the fact that all temporary and permanent changes to bodily structure and functions that the body is forced to undertake to protect itself from alcohol will alter its overall functioning. In the end, the liver and kidneys will be structurally and functionally altered due to the overwhelming burden that is placed upon them to eliminate the poison from the body.

Moreover, fetal blood alcohol concentration is the same as the blood alcohol concentration of the mother when she consumes an alcoholic beverage. The quantity of alcohol in her milk will depend on what she drank. If she only drank a small amount, it seems that the mammary glands can protect themselves.

"Furthermore, it seems that tissues are always affected in the same way by the same blood alcohol concentrations, regardless of the regularity of the person's alcohol consumption.

"In conclusion, what we mistakenly identify as tolerance is nothing more than the presence of a mechanism for delaying absorption and hastening elimination.
"In other words, the body will never learn to tolerate alcohol or any other poison.

"If the same blood alcohol concentration has the same effect on a drug addict's tissues as it does on a person who does not use drugs, this is certainly not a tolerance.

"The body has primary means of defense which it immediately calls to action as soon as a poison is consumed, and it also possesses secondary means of protection which it initiates when the ingestion of toxin becomes a regular occurrence.

"It is these secondary means of defense which are presumed to be tolerance. They are less violent, and therefore, they are less exhausting. By initiating these less tiring means of protection, the body can prolong its existence, despite its constant intoxication.

"Let's look at another example of a poison to which we pretend we are capable of adapting: arsenic. This moves us closer to coffee, tea, and tobacco. There again, we mistake pathological expediency for adaptation.

"When people take arsenic, we say that they are poisoning themselves. When drug users are deprived of their drugs, they rapidly develop the following symptoms:

- General malaise and indifference to those around them, anxiety.
- Loss of appetite, digestive troubles, heavy feeling in the stomach.
- Vomiting a runny liquid in the morning, accompanied by excessive salivation, heartburn, spastic contractions, and constipation.
- Shallow breathing.

"Those who quit arsenic experience gastric pains. Just as abandoning this poison is always followed by these morbid symptoms, the same symptoms always follow when stopping other drugs, including morphine, wine, tobacco, tea, coffee, cortisone, etc.

"As with all drugs, going back to drinking coffee will magically make all of the symptoms of withdrawal disappear.

"Thus, it's clear that drinkers do not return to their favorite poison because they want to – haven't we said that drugs have never engendered a desire to take them, such as opium in China, betel in India and loco in Peru – but to escape from the intolerable misery provoked by eliminating drugs, coffee, wine, tea, etc.

"Drug addicts, just like people who drink coffee, wine and the, think, based on their withdrawal experiences, that their poison is indispensable for their health! – Shelton

Headaches Are a Sign of Detoxification

Let us repeat one last time that when a person quits drinking coffee, smoking tobacco, etc., or, at the very least, goes for a period without these substances; the body begins a painful detoxification process, which is very difficult to endure. The person must be courageous to face it until all of the disagreeable symptoms come to an end before arriving at a poison—free state of well—being.

However, if the drug—addicted person or coffee drinker were to begin abusing their poison yet again, the body would stop its elimination process, thus inducing a false sense of well—being which perpetuates the endless, vicious cycle. It eventually leads to severe illnesses: blood disorders, leukemia, cirrhosis, nephritis, etc.

In the past, horses were given arsenic to fatten them, but as soon as the arsenic was taken away, the animal would become thin and wither away despite having an abundance of food at its disposal.

These horses were never able to return to their former appearance. This toxic method was employed to better sell the horses.

Why Do We Drink Coffee After We Wake Up?

Most people wake up with a foggy mind, heavy head and anxious, imprecise thoughts. In other words, most people wake up with the disagreeable of feeling that they aren't entirely awake, fit and full of energy. This is indicative of nocturnal elimination processes which have not yet finished. Thus, to halt it, we take a coffee to "wake up," as we so often say. Otherwise, how would we drive our car, go to work and focus on our tasks?

With coffee, the detoxification process stops the moment we wake up, and our mind once again becomes clear, and our normal concentration returns.

However, the health consequences of this delay are innumerable: blood disorders, nervous system disorders, liver, kidney and stomach afflictions, etc. Coffee is a drug, on par with any other drug. In its natural state, it is bitter. This should be enough to indicate to us that it is toxic.

How to Restore the Body's Natural Defenses

Our intestinal flora maintains our body's natural defenses. When this flora is healthy, food is properly digested, absorbed and assimilated. The bacteria in the intestines provide the body with the nutritive substances it requires to create red and white blood cells, which are indispensable for the body's natural defenses. This process is maintained by the body without any external assistance.

When we seek out external aids, such as antibiotics, to strengthen these defenses, we only weaken them and cause them to atrophy.

Therefore, those who wish to fortify these defenses need only work toward regenerating their precious intestinal flora.

What exactly is this flora?

It is made up of one hundred thousand billion beneficial microbes which form our body's perfect system of defense against infection.

Our microbial intestinal flora is the densest microbial grouping in the world, with most of them being useful to us. Its role has been demonstrated in:

- Intestinal transit,
- The speed at which cells are renewed,
- Protein synthesis,
- Water and ion absorption phenomena
- The creation of some rare vitamins, such as vitamin B12.
- Intestinal immunity
- Creating a barrier against attacks from other strains which might trigger infectious diseases.

These beneficial bacteria are capable of eliminating harmful bacteria, or at the very least prevent them from taking root within the body by limiting their ability to multiply and preventing them from increasing their population to the point of causing an infection.

Thus, as we have already said, this intestinal flora is made up of one hundred thousand billion bacteria. They maintain an incredible ecological equilibrium which, on its own, creates our body's system of defense against infection.

How to Restore the Intestinal Flora

I am often asked the following question:

"How can I restore my intestinal flora? Are there any natural products that can fortify it?"

To restore it, there are some steps which must be taken.

However, before considering these steps, let's look at two examples so that we may better understand the method that must be followed.

Tobacco and Bronchitis

A smoker suffers from chronic bronchitis stemming primarily from his or her use of tobacco. What should this person do to cure his or her bronchitis?

He must first stop using tobacco as it is the cause of their illness. In doing so, he will have completed 90% of the path to a "miraculous" bronchitis cure.

Should they be given a chemical medication or natural remedy? Not at all. Eliminating the cause is sufficient.

Can chemical or natural treatments (such as herbal tea, for example) speed up the healing process? No. These remedies only alleviate symptoms.

Alleviating symptoms is not equivalent to healing. In fact, this encourages the individual to keep smoking. It does not help at all with quitting tobacco. Instead, it creates obstacles for this elimination.

In reality, bronchitis itself is representative of the inflamed lungs attempting to rid themselves the toxic tobacco.

Hemorrhoids and Spices

Let's look at another, easily understandable example.

A person is suffering from hemorrhoids due to consuming spices and hot peppers (harissa, mustard, hot sauce, etc.). What should this person do to cure their hemorrhoids?

Should the patient be given an ointment for local use? Should they be given an oral medication? Should the patient be prescribed an herbal tea or plant extract?

All of these remedies aim to combat hemorrhoids without addressing their cause.

When your finger is burning because of exposure to fire, you just pull it away from the fire, and everything goes back to normal. In time, your finger will heal.

In this scenario, eliminating the cause is sufficient to cure the ailment. If we give the body enough time, it will repair itself.

In conclusion, eliminating spices from the diet would be enough to heal this patient's hemorrhoids.

What About Restoring a Destroyed Intestinal Flora?

To restore a gut flora that has been destroyed by chemical products, we must take a similar approach:

- First, we must eliminate whatever has destroyed the intestinal flora in the first place. This is 90% of the journey.

- Next, we must gradually stop eating foods which were never intended to be consumed by human beings. Consume only foods which are meant to be eaten by our species.

- Lastly, it's important to understand that there are no natural products or particular foods which can fortify and restore our intestinal flora. Those who suggest such products are only salespeople interested in their bottom line.

Eliminating the cause should be sufficient to return things to normal and restore the intestinal flora, so long we feed it natural nutrition.

Quickly washed, organic greens contain a multitude of bacteria which is indispensable for our flora. The same holds for yogurt and curdled milk.

> **Note from publisher**: Plant—based yogurts are advisable. Mosséri also mentioned that in one of his books.

CHAPTER 6: The Paradise Diet, According to Dr. Lovewisdom

> **Introduction from the publisher:**
>
> *I have decided to include this lesser—known chapter from one of Mosseri's books, because he had a particular fascination with the writings of Dr. Lovewisdom, a strange character who moved to Ecuador to live on a so—called "Paradise diet." However, having come across his writings myself and even exchanged some letters with him, I must say that Dr. Lovewisdom was a little "out there." Eventually, Mosséri settled for a more moderate position on nuts and seeds: eating them in moderation (about one ounce of nuts for non—athletic people, per day). Nonetheless, this chapter features some interesting gems of information. Lovewisdom may have been ahead of his time in realizing that high—protein foods stimulate growth. This could lead to some interesting conclusions in the treatment of cancer.*

Dr. J. Lovewisdom has led a campaign against eating various nuts for a long time.

Aphrodisiacs

"They disturb our sexual functions by provoking pathological phenomena, such as menstruation in women and involuntary emission of seminal fluids in men. As a result, self—control concerning reproductive functions becomes impossible, draining all energy and substance from the body.

"The role of seeds (grains and various nuts) in nature is as follows: they contain proteins intended to disseminate their species by producing plants which are similar to their progenitors. Thus, Nature did not intend for them to be eaten. Their role is rooted in reproduction.

"These reproductive substances lead to excessive reproduction in males. The poisons which allow for grains and various nuts to be digested have an irritating effect on sexual organs. The digestion of the concentrated proteins found in grains and nuts stimulates the sex glands, imposing a considerable amount of work on the body. Those who consume foods which are rich in proteins (meats, eggs, nuts, whole grains, dairy products) are very passionate.

A Foreign Substance

"All proteins are foreign substances in our body. The body must break them down into amino acids to neutralize them. Otherwise, they would poison the body to the point of death. Thus, the body breaks down the protein molecules not to appropriate the materials they contain – these materials are second—hand – but to protect itself against these foreign substances. The body renders them harmless by dismantling them. If these "food" proteins were to be injected directly into the blood, they would indeed be a dangerous poison. It's worth noting that snake venom is a protein.

Paranoia

"Uric acid is the byproduct of protein decomposition. It acidifies the body and irritates living cells. Through stimulation, this irritation creates a semblance of energy, but it is created at the cost of our vital forces, thus favoring illnesses. Consuming foods that are rich in proteins can give the impression of power, but it's always to the detriment of our nervous energy. Meat and various nuts are the foods which yield the most uric acid.

Enzyme Expenditure

"The digestion of grains and nuts is carried out by enzyme energy expenditure, but these foods don't have enzymes until they germinate. This is why our body has to use its enzymes, leading to useless energy expenditure.

Human Milk and Its Protein Content

"If there is one food that we can be sure is suited for human consumption, even if only for a limited time, it is without question human milk.

"Only fruits and vegetables have a composition which is similar to that of mother's milk. The percentage of proteins contained in mother's milk decreases after the birth of the newborn in the following way. (See the table at the top of the following page)

"Thus, we see that the protein composition of maternal milk declines, whereas the baby doubles its weight in only six months!

"This indicates that adults do not need foods containing more than 1% proteins. Fruits and vegetables fulfill this condition.

TABLE OF PROTEIN PERCENTAGES IN MILK

Five days after birth, milk contains..................... 5%
3—4 weeks after giving birth, it only contains....... 1.3%
7—8 weeks after giving birth, it only contains....... 1.2%

PERCENTAGE OF PROTEINS IN SOME FOODS

	FRESH	DRIED
Apples	0.4%	2%
Pears	0.6%	3.7%
Peaches	0.5%	3.9%
Melons	0.5%	6.2%
Oranges	0.9%	5%
Milk	1.4%	23%
Cheese	20% (approximately)	22%
Eggs (yolks)	12%	44%
Fish	18%	90%
Chicken	20%	75%
Dried peas	24%	28%
Wheat	14%	18%
Pecans	10%	12%
Almonds	19%	22%
Hazelnuts	16%	20%

Ratio of Proteins And Minerals

"We must consider the ratio of proteins to mineral salts in a given food. Once again, an ideal food should be similar in composition to human milk. If we consider the ratio of protein and calcium in peanuts, for example, we see that this nut contains 27% protein, and therefore, it should provide 1,080 mg of calcium. In reality, it only contains 74 mg. Similarly, meat contains 10 mg of calcium, but it should contain 720 mg.

"What do these numbers mean? It means that the body has to provide its alkaline mineral salts to neutralize the acidity of grains, which leads to demineralization.

"The same phenomenon happens with protein and phosphorus.

"Moreover, we know that an excess of protein can prevent calcium from being assimilated into the body.

Ratio of Water and Protein

"In addition to mineral ratios, an ideal food should also resemble the composition of mother's milk with regard to its ratio of water and protein. Human milk is 88% composed of living water, as indicated in the following table.

PERCENTAGE OF LIVING WATER IN FOODS

Food	Percentage
Human milk	88%
Juicy fruits and vegetables	90%
Cheese	70%
Eggs	70%
Meat	65%
Wheat	12%
Almonds	5%

"In short," concludes Lovewisdom, "only juicy fruits and vegetables are truly suitable for human consumption. They are very close in composition to maternal milk. Their living water 'washes away' each of our cells. They contain all of the minerals necessary for the development of the human body. They provide us with the solar energy that they have captured for themselves – they contain liquid sunlight! They don't foul the body with inert minerals that our body can't assimilate and other putrescible substances. They supply enzymes that are necessary for life. Because they don't irritate our sexual glands, they allow us to control our passion. In a word, they contain only virtues."

Infection and Cancer

A man named Dr. Lorinez has managed to reduce cancerous lumps in his patients by eliminating proteins from their diet. According to him, any cellular population which rapidly divides and grows will contain an enormous quantity of protein. Malignant tumors contain up to eleven times more protein than healthy tissues. Cancer which can no longer develop is cancer which can no longer kill.

"I've noticed," writes Lovewisdom, "that both old age and illness leave us feeling a so—called need for more protein. As we have come to see, this need is stimulated by outgrowths.

"After weeks or months, some cancer patients improve and can resume their normal activities. A woman who had been bedridden for a year from generalized cancer, whose doctor called her "more cancer than a person" was able to stand up, walk and return to a normal life after three months on a diet without proteins!"

A Sublime, Paradise Diet

Dr. Lovewisdom advocates for a diet composed exclusively of fruits and vegetables which is directed, he says,

"...against our lust for chaotic pleasure and against our absence of any willpower to change, to learn Dietary Science and Biological Chasteness, both of which build character.

"The low percentage of proteins contained in fruits, similar to that which is included in maternal milk, is most adapted to our body.

"The substance which is most adapted for transmitting genetic information – proteins – should not replace our supply of vital energies by provoking a deadly biological confrontation.

"Human beings do not have a grinding gizzard; therefore, they cannot grind grains in the way that Nature has ensured other species can.

"The threat of overpopulation which arises from the sexual stimulation provoked by a diet rich in nuts and grains could thus be resolved.

"A diet of seeds – grains and nuts – produces superfluous reproductive substances in the body which are contrary to the Laws of Nature. It causes sexual organs to become highly demanding, making us feel an incessant need.

"Dr. De la Torre, a well—known natural hygienist who ate 100 grams of various nuts nearly every day, died at the age of 72 despite his periodic fasts and naturally hygienic lifestyle. He didn't live any longer than all the people whose lifestyle he criticized."

I believe De la Torre suffered from tuberculosis. Thus, we can conclude that he would have died much younger than 72 years old had he lived off the same diet that much of the rest of the world consumes.

Dr. H.M. Shelton recommended that people eat an enormous 4 oz. (128 g.) serving of nuts each day. He was unaware of the fact that gorillas don't eat them, for this fact wasn't discovered until 1964 by Dr. Georges

Schaller, after having spent a year among gorillas in Africa.

Since then, many natural hygienists have reduced the daily recommended portion of various nuts to 3 oz. (90 g), but this amount is also too high. Instead, I recommend limiting them to one ounce per day (young athletes can eat two ounces).

Increased Innocence and Morality

"With a diet of raw foods, excluding grains, various nuts, and animal products, we are once again able to find our prepubescent sense of childlike innocence. We don't have to make the genetic sacrifice of millions of reproductive cells requiring the virtues of each cell of the parents to manifest identical heredity.

"The natural pattern of seeds and nuts is neither identical nor similar to human nutritive needs. On the contrary, it is entirely in opposition to these needs as we receive them through maternal milk and a diet of succulent fruits and raw vegetables.

"Furthermore, abnormal mental tendencies come from animal and plant—based proteins.

"Various nuts and grains cause sensual pleasure, just like meats and other foods with high concentrations of proteins. This only causes the body to degenerate.

"A diet whose protein content is similar to that of milk is a clean diet that will lead to mental equilibrium, healthy behavior, balanced reasoning and a moral life.

"Let us now look at what happens when we eat fruit. They contain very little protein because they do not need to transmit the genetic information any more than the morphology – that is, the strength and design – of plans can be of any use to human morphology for its hereditary traits.

"Moreover, the enzymes which accompany food elements allow for them to be almost instantaneously assimilated with the lowest possible amount of wear and tear to the body's economic integrity.

"Plant and animal genetic information and substance is not transferable to human energy.

"Therefore, a deadly conflict and natural antagonism follow.

"The body is then obligated to dismantle the proteins into amino acids with high gastric acidity, thus causing the acidic saturation that Dr. Cril and many others believe to be the cause of old age and death.

"It has also been observed that aside from heat and cooking, enzymes can also be destroyed by acidity. In this case, an acidifying diet can ruin enzymes, leading to a massive loss of energy and substance.

"Plant enzymes initiate their growth through germination and are not capable of making it possible for the substances contained in grains to be assimilated by humans.

"In 1942, researcher A.I. Virtane showed that living plant proteins are, for the most part, enzymes which, in living cells, are found separate from their respective substrates.

"From the very moment that the cells are crushed (when chewing, for example) the enzymes are freed, entering into contact with their respective substrates within the mass of chewed food.

"As a result, enzymatic decomposition processes can begin in the mouth. A portion of this newly freed matter can have a significant physiological impact.

"This physiologically active matter which comes to the enzymatic processes affecting the chewed food is then reabsorbed in the intestines and arrives in tissue cells via the blood along with all other nutritive matters.

"We don't completely understand the physiological action of the active matter, but we can nevertheless be sure of the considerable impact it has on the body's metabolism.

"Since all enzymes are denatured and rendered inactive at temperatures varying from 60 C and 100 C, no enzymatic reaction takes place when the body absorbs cooked foods." – Professor Henning Karstrom from the University of Helsinki. – The Natural Life, No. 20.

Biological Transmutations

"The body must produce its enzymes or create special, adapted enzymes which are "customized," so to speak, to accomplish a specific task, but this causes the body to lose a considerable amount of energy, thus leading to exhaustion.

"However, if the body can create special enzymes when they're needed, it can surely create any protein it needs to build cells from the air we breathe and the amino acids in food."

Biological transmutations can also explain many things in this unexplored field. When the body needs proteins, it creates them in its intestinal flora from the elements that it already possesses.

Researcher and chemist Louis Kervran found that chickens which had been fed a diet devoid of all calcium nevertheless continued to lay eggs as if nothing were wrong. We know that eggshells contain calcium, so what happened? What is the mystery? They merely had to transmute the sodium, magnesium, and phosphorus contained in their food into calcium within their intestinal flora.

This is nature's way of carrying out humanity's ancient dream of somehow turning lead into gold.

Misguided Instincts

"You ask me," Dr. Lovewisdom wrote me, "why we shouldn't eat seeds – grains nuts, and seeds.

"When I was a young boy, I thought that the only food nature intended for us to eat fruit.

"I do not believe in Darwin's theory of evolution," continues Dr. Lovewisdom."

"I do not believe that everything evolved from chaos and confusion. My Universe is one of Intelligent Order. All of Creation has a purpose – Nature is guided by Intelligence for Biological Goals.

"Seeds were made for the reproduction of each species, each within its genre. They were not made to become food for superior beings who can reason and act in harmony with Nature's design and plan."

I think that the more structurally complex a being is, the more it becomes specialized in the materials it uses. It is no longer able to use materials such as they are presented through plant—based and animal proteins: it must make its proteins.

Monkeys and birds obey their instincts, not their intelligence. I do not think that they are mistaken, as Dr. Lovewisdom seems to suggest, but for human beings, intelligence appears to have replaced our misguided and lost instincts, and unfortunately, this intelligence is not fully developed and is not blossoming in all people.

It's better to count on the instincts of primates when deciding how to feed ourselves than to rely on the instincts of more evolved human beings.

"When necessary (when fruit is lacking), we can turn to all kinds of vegetables and root vegetables (like potatoes) before resorting to consuming grains. Roots are foods which do not contain reproductive substances.

"In times of famine, animals and humans sometimes begin to eat the earth, thinking it can nourish them.

"You say that birds eat grains, and monkeys eat nuts. However, monkeys also sometimes eat eggs which are indicative of how intelligent they are."

Chickens Made Carnivorous

"To produce large numbers of eggs," continues Dr. Lovewisdom, "farmers have turned to a diet of grains for feeding their chickens. However, this is the same diet that we give to nations who are stricken by famine while simultaneously teaching them about birth control! Alas, the only result is population growth, pollution, poverty, war, and suffering. Feeding the world with reproductive food substances is the cause of all this overpopulation.

"The same is true for individual humans, on a microcosmic level, and all of humanity collectively on a macrocosmic level. In fact, the more we introduce these reproductive substances into, the more, the more we are encouraging wild growth and protrusions, such as cancers, bacterial outgrowths, and viruses."

When Lovewisdom wrote these lines, farmers were stuffing their chickens with grains so that they would produce the most eggs. In Nature, chickens, or rather, the birds from which they descend, search for their food – grains, fruits, greens, – and therefore, they are active and only eat what little they find. Chickens raised by farmers, on the other hand, produce many eggs because they are inactive and are stuffed with food.

Nowadays, things have changed once again. Chickens are now raised industrially and fed with slaughterhouse waste. Their food has become meat—based, and thus, chickens have become carnivorous – they were initially granivorous – and they now lay more eggs, but they are plagued with dangerous bacteria, such as salmonella, in their intestinal flora. Their eggs are simultaneously infected with this salmonella. As time goes on, eating eggs becomes more and more of a dangerous affair.

In France, importing eggs from Great Britain is prohibited, but we refuse to recognize that in France, our chickens will be affected by this same bacteria sooner or later.

A Sublime, Paradise Diet

"In short," concludes Lovewisdom, "we have discovered a new science which has the power to eliminate menstruation in women and cause the involuntary loss of seminal fluid due to leaking in men.

"Animal passions are thus pushed aside in human beings to the extent that he can live on an elevated spiritual plane rather than being a slave to his lust and desires."

"Blood flows undisturbed," André Gide would say, (Cellars of the Vatican), but not without heat.

"Of course, people are not born as masters of the self, aspiring to spiritual goals, peace, and happiness. The average person will instead follow in the footsteps of beasts, monkeys, birds, and pigs as guides for becoming an ideal human.

"Darwin created a doctrine adapted to the fetishist ideas and animal passion of his followers.

"You can see the result of this in questions of morality and immorality. Animal sexuality and ideas are widespread, just like human deaths in wars, abortion, famine, etc.

> **Final comments from the publisher:**
>
> *It's clear here that while Mosséri translated this passionate pamphlet from Lovewisdom, he didn't believe every word of it. There's more than just a small undertone of religious fanaticism. That being said, Lovewisdom was on to something, with some of his affirmations. There's no credible reason to eliminate nuts entirely from the diet, but at the same time, a low-protein diet of fruits and greens can be incredibly useful in some circumstances.*

CHAPTER 7: How to Find Your Way Among Various Dietary Systems

If a beginner were to buy several different books about alternative medicine, they would quickly start to feel lost while reading through all the contradictions presented by various naturopathic authors.

Before we tackle these contradictions, let's look at a few rough vocabulary definitions for terms that are necessary to understanding trends among alternative medicine's numerous (and sometimes opposing) systems.

Fruitarian. Someone who only eats fruits (including various nuts, tomatoes, cucumbers, and peppers, which are also fruits).

Vegetarian. Someone who does not eat meat, though they may eat animal products (milk, dairy products, cheeses, eggs, honey). They eat grains, fruits, vegetables, various nuts and animal byproducts. The term "vegetarian" is the most well—known and also the best. We will see why a bit later. A pure vegetarian is a Natural Hygiene practitioner.

Raw Foodist. — Those who follow this diet only eat raw foods.

"Instincto" Instinctotherapy practitioners, sometimes called instinctos, eat everything raw, and they rely on their instinct – that is, their sense of smell – to choose their foods. They may also eat raw meat and raw fish.

Vegan. Someone who only eats plant foods and does not eat animal byproducts. Their diet includes grains and various nuts; their diet excludes dairy products and eggs.

Naturopath. Practitioners who refuse to take chemical medications, instead of using "natural" medicine to treat their ailments. These natural alternatives include clay, water, foods, compresses, chiropractic medicine, acupuncture, massages, herbal teas, etc. They aim to eliminate their symptoms with the help of these remedies.

Natural Hygienist. — People who are mindful of all things healthy, who care for the ill and who refuse to use any form of medicine, even if it's natural. They focus on eliminating the cause of their ailments and fasting. They don't use herbal teas, massages, sitz baths, acupuncture, chiropractic medicine, clay, hydrotherapy, psychoanalysis, drinking urine, deep breathing, forced breathing or any other artificial means of alleviating symptoms.

Macrobiotics. This Japanese system recommends following a diet based on brown rice, with added salt.

Shelton uses the word "frugivore," but his definition of the term includes vegetables and greens.

Some vegetables – tomatoes, peppers, cucumbers, etc. – are also fruits, botanically speaking, because they have a flower. Greens and roots, such as carrots and potatoes, are not fruits.

The word "vegetarian" should encompass many of these other terms and should not in any way include bread and grains because they are not naturally consumed by human beings and cannot be consumed raw. They can only be consumed when they have germinated because the starch is transformed into easily digested carbohydrates.

As for the term "vegan," which includes plants while excluding animal byproducts, it's redundant. Consuming these animal foods is not natural. Milk should, according to Nature, be consumed by children. Cheeses are not natural. Eggs are stolen from the chickens to whom they belong just as honey is stolen from bees.

Furthermore, all of these dietary systems allow for the excessive consumption of nuts and seeds. Since we avoid consuming large quantities of nuts and there is no term which adequately encapsulates our diet, we have used the word "hygienist" or "Natural Hygienist" to this end. The word "vegetarian" can also be used, but only in the purest and most hygienic sense of the word.

To summarize, humans who follow an enlightened, Natural Hygiene diet are vegetarians, though they are the purest form of vegetarians.

The word "vegetarian" should only include foods which were intended to be consumed by our species. Therefore, if we concern ourselves with what is healthy and unhealthy, a vegetarian diet should automatically exclude animal foods and grains, without having to indicate this exclusion. We may also call this "pure vegetarianism."

A vegetarian who eats cheese, many nuts, eggs, and bread is an undiscerning and impure vegetarian who consumes foods which are not intended for human beings. This vegetarian is not concerned with what is healthy or unhealthy. These vegetarians only worry about not causing animals to suffer by killing them.
A vegan who eats excessive amounts of almonds and peanuts with little regard for the types of plants they consume is not someone who is looking to improve their health.

There are only concerned with not stealing from animals.

Instinctotherapy practitioners would have us rely on our sense of smell to guide us in our (always raw) food choices, even if that choice were meat or fish. Some also recommend a plant—based laxative (cassia) after each meal! Because our instincts are so depraved, we cannot rely on them to guide us to choose healthy foods. We can be attracted by tasty food, even after having eaten the point satiation.

Grain—Based Macrobiotic Diets

We have already said that while humans have consumed meat for centuries and centuries, the human body has still not evolved past its vegetarian characteristics.

The same can be said for the grain—based diet that humans have consumed for thousands of years. This diet of bread – or rice, in Asian countries – has not led to any anatomical or physiological changes in the human body which would lead it to be classified as granivorous. We still lack a grinding gizzard for hard, tough seeds. Our salivary glands still don't secrete enough ptyalin to process the large quantities of starch that these grains contain.

Human Beings: a Single Species

Some dietary systems would have people change their diet by their climate, habits, race, origin, level of health, etc.

"Human beings," notes Shelton, "are only one species. We can draw a general dietary conclusion and apply it to all people, regardless of where in the world they live.

"The structural anatomical differences and functional physiological differences which would be required to classify some human beings as carnivorous while classifying others as frugivorous would be so great that it would be impossible for these two groups of people to belong to a single species. Such variations are simply not found among human beings."

Thus, the diet which is best for human beings must be that which is best for all human beings. In reality, we all have the same anatomical organs which perform the same physiological functions.
We can see the error committed by those who believe humans should change their diet to suit their climate, habits, race, and region.

In fact, the Eskimo are not accustomed to consuming fish any more than the Chinese are accustomed to eating rice. Europeans are not accustomed to eating wine and meat, and Egyptians are not accustomed to eating dried beans.

The variations occurring in all these populations are pathological changes. Their structure remains vegetarian. They have not developed anatomical and physiological structures which would make them carnivorous or granivorous (i.e., eating seeds and grains).

The only variations that Nature allows for any given species pertain to the quantity of food to be eaten, not the type of food. It's possible to individualize a diet, but it must remain within certain general rules.

Nevertheless, we must emphasize a few details. There is no doubt that in the case of chronic illness, the patient must eat more vegetables than fruits.

Moreover, some people have food sensitivities. For example, their body might come to digest certain foods poorly, but these sensitivities can usually be overcome through fasting.

Lastly, imported foods are perfectly acceptable for hygienists; it is not necessary to strictly adhere to only locally grown foods.

Is Cooking All That Harmful?

Let's talk briefly about cooking foods. Some people are vehemently against cooked foods, including a fair amount of Natural Hygienists.

Toward the end of the 1930s, Hans Eppinger (of Vienna) made the particularly remarkable observation that raw, vegetarian foods considerably improved the diffusion of nutritive materials and oxygen from the capillary vessels to the cells.

It is for the same reason that, in reverse, carbon dioxide and waste is guided from the cells to the capillaries.

Therefore, it follows that raw foods encourage both nutrition and detoxification while cooked foods inhibits these processes.

Thus, the body may not be adapted to consuming cooked foods.

Nevertheless, when we look at a tribe in New Guinea whose diet was 90% composed of sweet potatoes cooked on hot stones and consider how healthy they are, we have to hesitate before incriminating cooking as the primary cause of all our health problems.

Instead, we should say that there is cooking and then there's *cooking*. Cooking foods at high temperatures, such as the heat we see in ovens, or frying them in butter and oil cannot be compared to the partial cooking when foods are cooked rapidly (without the addition of fats, at a temperature which remains below 100 C). The latter cannot be too harmful to our health.

We cannot highlight such an innocuous form of cooking as a cause for illness while we commit much more serious mistakes like drinking coffee, eating nuts or cheese or just staying up late at night and overworking without taking a moment to rest.

This is the problem with many of these dietary systems. They emphasize unimportant details and remain silent on the grave errors.

CHAPTER 8: Table Of Comparative Anatomy And Physiology

CARNIVORES	OMNIVORES	HERBIVORES	ANTHROPODIAL MONKEYS	HUMANS
Zonary placenta	Cotyledonary placenta	Cotyledonary placenta	Discoidal placenta	Discoidal placenta
4 feet	4 feet	4 feet	2 hands and 2 feet	2 hands and 2 feet
Claws	Hooves	Cloven hooves	Flat nails	Flat nails
Tail	Tail	Tail	No tail	No tail
Eyes look sideways	Eyes look sideways	Eyes look sideways	Eyes look forward	Eyes look forward
Skin does not have pores	Skin has some pores	Skin has some pores (excluding pachyderms, such as elephants)	Millions of pores	Millions of pores
Undeveloped incisors	Very well-developed incisors		Well-developed incisors	Well-developed incisors
Sharp molars	Folded molars		Dull molars	Dull molars
Dental formula: 5 to 8.1.6.1.5 to 8 5 to 8.1.6.1.5 to 8	Dental formula: 8.1.2 to 3.1.8 8.1.2 to 3.1.8	Dental formula: 6.0.0.6 6.1.6.1.6	Dental formula: 5.1.4.1.5 5.1.4.1.5	Dental formula: 5.1.4.1.5 5.1.4.1.5
Small salivary glands	Well-developed salivary glands	Well-developed salivary glands	Well-developed salivary glands	Well-developed salivary glands

Acidic urine and saliva	Acidic urine and saliva	Alkaline urine and saliva	Alkaline urine and saliva	Urine and saliva should normally be alkaline
Tongue for shredding	Smooth tongue	Smooth tongue	Smooth tongue	Smooth tongue
Nipples on abdomen	Nipples on abdomen	Nipples on abdomen	Mammary glands on chest	Mammary glands on chest
Simple stomach	Round stomach	Stomach with 3 chambers (in camels and certain ruminants, there are 4 chambers)	Stomach with duodenum (like a 2nd stomach)	Stomach with duodenum (like a 2nd stomach)
Intestinal tract that is 3x as long as the body	Intestinal tract that is 10x as long as the body	Intestinal tract length varies by species. In general, it is 10x as long as the body	Intestinal tract is 12x as long as the body	Intestinal tract is 12x as long as the body
Smooth colon	Smooth, convoluted intestinal tract	Smooth, convoluted intestinal tract	Convoluted colon	Convoluted colon
Live off animal flesh	Live off animal flesh, carrion and plants	Live off grass and plants	Live off fruits and greens	Should live off fruits and greens

CHAPTER 9: Comparative Anatomy And Physiology

Vocabulary

Before studying the table we have just seen in the previous chapter, let's take a look at a few words and how we will be using them in our discussion.

The word *frugivore* is used to designate those who exclusively eat fruits. No animal on earth is 100% *frugivorous*.

The word vegetarian is used to designate those who eat plant foods. This should exclude grains (as they are not edible in their natural state) and animal products, such as dairy, cheese and the eggs that we steal from chickens. In common parlance, the word vegetarian is used to refer to those who eat everything except meat.

The word vegan, which excludes consumption of all animal products, is redundant.

Lastly, the term *hygienist* (or an enlightened vegetarian) refers to those who take Natural Hygiene into account, refusing to eat large quantities of nuts (one ounce per day is good).

Human Beings Are Vegetarian; They Are Neither Carnivorous Nor Granivorous

The Table of Comparative Anatomy and Physiology presented in the previous chapter was taken from an article written by Dr. Shelton in his Hygienic Review. That table was reproduced from Dr. Emmet Densmore's 1892 work, *How Nature Cures*.

This table, in turn, was improved upon by Densmore himself after being pulled from a version that was initially published in German by author Gustav Schlickeysen in his work, "Fruit and Bread." This original version of the table did not contain the column detailing the anatomical and physiological characteristics of herbivores. Dr. Densmore himself added this column.

An intelligent person need only examine the 17 anatomical and physiological differences outlined in this table to understand that human beings, as descendants of primates, should be classified as vegetarians. This means that humans should eat plants – fruits, greens, and vegetables – in the same state that Nature has provided them. This excludes grains because although they come from plants, they are not edible when raw.

Another consideration is the fact that while bananas are technically plants which are pleasant to see, smell and taste, enlightened Natural Hygienists refuse to eat them. This is because gorillas refuse to eat them, and their instinct is undoubtedly more reliable than our own. Prunes, apricots, and pineapples are acceptable, despite any reservations which Shelton may have had.

> **Note from publisher:** Mosséri eventually went back on his anti—banana stance, stating that they needed to be very ripe to be consumed.

The Placenta

The first row in the table designates the type of placenta possessed by species within the category in question. Professor Huxley considered this to be the best way to classify a given species. From this data, we see that humans fall definitively within the vegetarian category. Read more to this end in Professor Thomas Henry Huxley's work, *Man's Place in Nature*.

Teeth

Let's move on and discuss tooth shape, which is mentioned very briefly in the table.

It's universally acknowledged that tooth shape is hugely important when classifying an animal. We can see from just a quick glance at this table that great apes come between human beings and carnivores, not the other way around. This indicates that human beings are the archetype of vegetarians.

The average reader, lacking the scientific training required to understand such detailed research, need only understand the most simple and most striking detail: this is a question of the shape of our teeth.

Open your dog or cat's mouth and look at their long, tapered, razor—sharp canine teeth, capable of interlocking in two opposing grooves on each side of the jaw. Take a look at their range of incisors as well. We find them between the aforementioned canine teeth. You can also see the two series of teeth behind these incisors which close on one another like a double—toothed saw; they're for cutting and tearing.

Next, compare the animal's teeth with the structure and arrangement of your teeth. They're completely different.

If you try to force your cat to make a lateral grinding motion with its lower jaw, the cat will tell you, in its way, that the movement is not natural.

The same is true for greyhounds and bulldogs.

All of these observations are both general and universal; they are neither accidental nor exceptional. In fact, there is no carnivorous animal on earth which lacks these long, tapering and razor—sharp canine teeth. Furthermore, no carnivore is capable of moving its jaw laterally.

Similarly, there are no vegetarian animals or herbivores which have the canine teeth we have just described. They all possess molars and the capacity to move their lower jaw laterally.

Therefore, it seems evident that we should classify human beings as vegetarians. Our teeth are made for chewing up fruits and vegetables, whereas carnivores, such as dogs, have teeth designed for tearing through meat.

Mammary Grands And Sex

It's also important to study the arrangement of an animal's mammary glands. As a general rule, carnivores have mammary glands arranged in rows along each side of their abdomen and chest. Herbivores (except for elephants) have mammary glands between their hindquarters.

Apes and humans, on the other hand, have two breasts, one on each side of their chest.

The structural arrangement and location of sexual organs are equally crucial for classifying various species.

Humans Are Not Predators

Even a child can easily see that humans are not predators, for they do not have the characteristics that a carnivorous lifestyle requires.

The more we study the structure of the human body, the more we can see that it resembles that of higher primates (who are vegetarians), as opposed to that of omnivores and carnivores, which sustain themselves by preying.

Sharp fangs, ferocious claws, and other physical characteristics make carnivores ideal predators. Human beings, on the other hand, are not equipped to lead a predatory lifestyle.

Even cave dwellers (who, let's not forget, were exceptions to the rule) lived in groups and fed from dead or dying animals that were already in a somewhat advanced state of decay. They scavenged these corpses because they didn't have the means to hunt and kill prey themselves.

If humans had been entirely carnivorous, they would have indeed been the most miserable and poorly equipped species in all of nature, regarding their ability to obtain their meat—based food.

It's curious that followers of instinctotherapy have been misled in their observations and reasoning about our original diet. In fact, even if cave dwellers did eat meat, that still isn't representative of the majority of mankind, who lived in tropical regions where succulent fruits and vegetables would grow spontaneously.

Lost in the cold and inhumane climates of Europe, famished and trying to survive, what else could the unfortunate cavemen do? Is that the diet that instinctotherapy theorists would have us establish as an example to follow?

Cave dwellers were nothing more than miserable saprophytes and street—sweepers, on par with vultures, jackals, and crows, seeking out decaying animal carcasses that had already been killed or that had died from illness. With their bare hands, they could only hope to trap insects, small animals like mice and lizards or steal from bird nests.

However, as is the case elsewhere in Nature, this kind of nutrition can only lead to the stagnation and degeneration of the species in question. It ultimately leads to the species' extinction, following numerous serious illnesses.

When biologists talk about a species' extinction, they voluntarily skip over the intermediary stages in which the species becomes ill and begins to degenerate and simply present the extinction as though it happened abruptly. It reminds me of the way the media announces a famous person's death. They recount the person's life, their works, and their accomplishments, and then, quite suddenly, they announce that the person has died. They just skip over the years of suffering and illness that the person had to endure before dying in agony. If they were to address it, the public would want to know why the person had suffered so much and why nothing was done to eliminate the cause of their suffering. No, we prefer to say that they were sick for some time. Briefly, they battled courageously, and then, they passed away. Wouldn't have been more courageous to stop consuming coffee, wine, tobacco and other poisons?

In short, it's impossible to imagine that any such carnivorous ancestors could have led their species to progress in any way. Instead, we should talk about their regression.

The Mouth

Throughout the animal kingdom, mouths evolve by the nature of the foods they consume, as this is how the food is obtained.

If the animal uses its hands to collect food, such as to pick an apple and bring the apple to its mouth, for example, the mouth doesn't need to be specially designed to obtain food. In these animals, the mouth doesn't need to extend away from the face.

On the contrary, animals that use their mouth to collect food require a long muzzle which opens far away from their eyes. These animals need lips and a long row of teeth to grasp their food. For example, look at grazing herbivores like horses, cows, gazelles, etc. They have a long face and a mouth that protrudes quite far away from their eyes.

Although carnivores use their forelegs to a certain extent to obtain food, they rely on their mouth both to grasp and kill their prey.

Lastly, primates use their hands to secure their food, thus rendering a specialized mouth useless to this end. They only need their simple hands to collect food and bring it to their mouths.

Now, let's consider for a moment that human beings use their hands more than other primates when preparing their foods to be eaten. In fact, other primates use their teeth for food preparation, such as to shell nuts. Thus, human hands can accomplish tasks which require the use of a muzzle for carnivores, omnivores, and herbivores. Humans do not belong to the same category as them.

Moreover, it's impossible for us to conceive of a world in which human beings stick out their nose like an animal, using their sense of smell to inspect every new object they encounter. Followers of instinctotherapy are once again mistaken.

In fact, human beings, like lemurs, rely more on their hands than their sense of smell. Even elephants smell their food with their long nose to separate what they want to eat from what they refuse because their anatomy doesn't allow for them to quickly grasp food in their mouth as a dog or cow might. This doesn't mean that humans and lemurs never smell their food, but we aren't meant to seek out food with our mouth.

As for granivorous animals, they use their beak to peck at seeds; this is also not the case for human beings. Instead, we use our hands to pick fruits and vegetables. Human beings are not granivorous and should not consume grains.

The Liver

The perfect harmony and adaptation of each organ about the function for which it was created reigns supreme in Nature. We find that the same is true when we examine the interior regions of our body to study the structure and function of our organs.

Relative to the body's overall size, carnivores possess a much larger liver than that of apes and humans. This allows them to process high—protein foods fully.

From an anatomical point of view, aside from everything that we've been saying rather succinctly, an entire book could be written on this subject without even exhausting everything that can be said. This would prove beyond a shadow of a doubt that human beings are vegetarians, not carnivores.

I don't understand how followers of instinct therapy, who see no problem with eating meat and fish, were able to be led astray in this field. Why did they close their eyes to these indisputable facts and refuse to see that cave dwellers, whose sense of taste was depraved, were forced to eat rotten meat to survive the cold and famine? Why did they elevate cave dwellers as an example to be followed, labeling their carnivorous ways as humanity's original diet, when it was a diet which that of a minuscule fraction of human beings, the majority of whom lived in tropical regions where succulent fruits and vegetables grew naturally?

> *Note from the publisher: Although instinctotherapy is not a popular diet anymore, the Paleo diet is. Almost everything that Mosséri mentions about instinctive eating could apply to the more recent Paleo craze.*

Position Of the Jaw

Note that in carnivorous animals – lions, tigers, wolves, dogs, cats – the lower jaw protrudes outward in front of the upper jaw.

Vegetarians like sheep and cows, on the other hand, have the opposite jaw structure.

In human beings and monkeys, the lower jaw lies behind the superior jaw with a few rare exceptions where we see the opposite arrangement. In these cases, the anomaly is clear. There are probably several causes for this anomaly: cross—strains, children of parents who are too close genetically, such as in the case of incest.

Facial Resemblance

How does this table of comparative anatomy and physiology lead us to conclude that in general, human beings are vegetarians? By solely comparing the similar structures and particularities among diverse animals, we can see the behaviors and dispositions which align similar animals into a single category. This doesn't mean that if a single human being were to be designed in a certain way or presented some particular, individual characteristic which resembled some other animal that he should be classified as belonging to the same animal with whom he shares some vague resemblance.

For example, a human being whose face has a vague, imaginary resemblance to that of a mouse should never be classified as a mouse. In fact, the deformations which lead to such similarities are not valid criteria for any legitimate, meaningful classification.

Let's look at another example. If the lower jaw projects outward in front of the upper jaw in a particular human being, this human should not be classified as a carnivore due to this trait, for it is a deformation.

A generic human being must be compared with a generic vegetarian, generic carnivore, generic herbivore, and generic omnivore. Individual variations are not a basis for correct general classifications. Moreover, facial resemblances alone are not sufficient for establishing a global classification.

Comparative anatomy and physiology study humanity as a whole – not a single individual but the entire species – to yield an accurate classification.

In short, all throughout Nature, we find well—defined adaptations between various organisms and the different foods they are intended to eat. Human beings, whom we mustn't forget are just another kind of animal, are not an exception to this rule.

It would seem, it is sometimes said, that carnivores and omnivores are not as well—adapted to their source of food as herbivores and vegetarians are. The former, being far from their original standards and with the positive and negative compensations they have had to undergo to adapt to illegitimate foods, have not adapted perfectly. For believers, the Bible indicates that all animals were originally vegetarian. Should we see all of this in philosophical speculation or physiological realities?

Birds and Reptiles

In their stomachs, birds have a grinding gizzard to grind up the raw grains they peck. To this end, they swallow stones, even needles, to help them in this endeavor. Human beings do not have this grinding gizzard. Therefore, a smart mind invented the grinding wheel, but Nature does not allow imitation without reacting. In fact, digestive juices, not adapted to digest grains, are far from being able to process them.

Falcons, eagles and other carnivorous birds have talons which are in sharp contrast with the feet of granivorous birds.

Also striking is the strong, curved upper mandible which is longer and folds back upon the lower jaw in these same carnivorous birds. They have the anatomical equipment that their predatory life requires, whereas granivorous birds lack these characteristics.

As for reptiles, we see similar characteristics, as with carnivorous fish and insects.

Human Beings Are Classified As Vegetarians

All throughout nature, animals have different physical characteristics for gathering food following their dietary practices.

Humans are the only exception! Our dietary practices are incredibly varied, yet according to our fundamental nature and all evidence, they should be restricted to those of higher primates – that is, vegetarian.

Alas, how do we explain this disconnect between human nature and abnormal human practices? There indeed must have been a moment at which we veered off the path from our primitive norms in favor of following a diet that goes against our anatomical, physiological and psychological nature.

Biologists maintain that human beings should be classified among monkeys and apes due to our physical structure and the way in which our brain is formed. They also recognize the fact that human beings are radically different from carnivores in several significant ways.

Nowadays, since we teach biology in our schools, no one can pretend that human beings are similar to carnivorous dogs; instead, we are more closely related to great apes, being the archetype of primates. This is every bit as true for our digestive tract as it is for the rest of our anatomical structures.

Two General Principles Of Biology

The following two principals were outlined by Sylvester Graham, one of the foremost hygienists of the 19th century.

There is a defined relationship between an animal's physical constitution and their natural source of food.

The food to which any animal – human or otherwise – is naturally and fundamentally adapted is the food which will best serve their highest biological, physiological and psychological needs.

The logical deduction which arises from this second proposition is as follows:

The more that human beings distance themselves from Nature's standards in their food habits, the more their health and happiness will be affected by this decision.

It isn't sufficient to simply think that we're happy eating whatever delicious meals come our way while fooling our sense of taste with unhealthy artifice. We can also find happiness by taking drugs or smoking!

Illness, deformation, and degeneration are the prices that human beings pay for distancing themselves from Nature's standards in every aspect of their life, not limited to food practices.

The universality of this degeneration and illness is scathing proof that human beings are a fallen species.

"Even the presence of doctors and healers among us is an anomaly which comes from our distance from Nature's normal paths," wrote Shelton.

Comparative Physiology

We have now studied a bit of comparative anatomy for the main categories of animals, but comparative physiology is also fascinating, as we will soon see. It also leads us to maintain that human beings are vegetarians rather than carnivores or granivores.

Anatomical structure and physiological structure are so interlocked, so very linked and integrated, that, in the past, there have been debates as to whether "the organ determines its function or the function designs the organ."

This correspondence between organs and structures with their physiological functions as a means to classify humans as vegetarians are, therefore, wholly justified.

Here again, followers of instinctotherapy, who suggest eating raw meat, got it wrong. How have they been able to ignore such scientific and biological considerations only to hold on to humanity's depraved instincts as a means of justifying meat consumption?

Ptyalin

The salivary secretions of carnivores do not contain ptyalin as this enzyme aids in breaking down starches.

Herbivores and primates, on the other hand, do possess this enzyme which is significant from a physiological point of view because it demonstrates beyond a shadow of a doubt that these animals can digest a specific type of food, whereas carnivores are adapted to a different kind of food.

Nevertheless, the quantity of ptyalin secreted by primates is low when compared to the amount secreted by granivores. This shows that primates are not equipped to process foods that are too starchy, such as grains and bread.

Various roots, such as potatoes, carrots, and rutabagas, are low enough in starches that the salivary glands of humans and primates can process them.

Thus, from an anatomical and physiological point of view, the differences between human beings, carnivores and granivores are great enough that they justify classifying human beings in a different category than these other animals.

Uricase And Uric Acid

Uricase is an enzyme possessed by some (though not all) animals, according to Darland's *American Medical Dictionary*. It is a catalyzer in the complex transformation of uric acid into "allantoin."

However, with a few exceptions, it seems that this enzyme is not found in primates, whereas it is found in insects and a breed of Dalmatians that excrete uric acid like human beings.

In animals which possess uricase, 80—90% of all uric acid is oxidized and transformed into allantoin and carbon dioxide. Uric acid byproducts have not been discovered in human beings. This acid was the last step in the disintegration of this poison coming from protein metabolism.

Finally, it is believed that the reduction of uric acid and its decomposition into allantoin happens primarily in the liver.

"Allantoin is 250 times more soluble than uric acid." This means that animals which possess this enzyme can eliminate a more considerable amount of uric acid than those who do not possess it. When taking into consideration the fact that consuming meat produces an abundance of uric acid, we can easily understand why carnivores can fully process their meat—based diet. This is what makes uricase interesting.

This physiological difference distinguishes vegetarians from other categories of animals. In fact, on the one hand, vegetarians possess ptyalin, whereas, on the other hand, carnivores possess uricase. Uricase allows the liver in animals who possess it to carry out a function which the livers of primates cannot undertake.

The Digestive Tract

The various digestive tract lengths of the various categories of animals allow for different types of digestion to be carried out in each.

Physiologists have noted the length of the intestines in herbivores, as well as the presence of two or three pockets where food can stay for a rather long time. They have also emphasized that carnivores have rather short intestines which lack these pockets.

Granivores, for their part, have a grinding gizzard which doesn't exist in carnivores and herbivores.

Therefore, it's clear that the digestive function of these various categories of animals is not the same due to the different kinds of food on which they subsist.

There are also relevant differences in their digestive secretions and enzymes, which are necessary for the different types of diets these animals consume. The absence of ptyalin in carnivores and the reduced or absent flow of uricase in vegetarians — these are only some of these enzymatic differences.

Pavlov, the great Russian physiologist, has also found that carnivores have almost no ability to break down starches. Furthermore, in the wild, a carnivorous would include a variety of pre—digested sugars.

"If a normal primate diet contains more sugar than starch, this sugar is nevertheless not always presented in a form which doesn't require digestion. For this reason, they are equipped with pancreatic and intestinal enzymes which are capable of reducing these complex sugars into monosaccharides, but since their diet also contains starches, their saliva is capable of transforming starches into sugars."

"While the digestive tract of primates resembles that of a carnivore more than that of a herbivore, it is equipped to process a type of food which a carnivore's digestive tract would be incapable of processing." Shelton

Canine Teeth And Assumptions About Their Origin

We have emphasized the fact that function and structure are both important in our quest to classify the human diet.

It's worth noting, nevertheless, that while humans do possess "canine teeth," they don't serve the same purpose as those which dogs and cats have, without even beginning to talk about lions and tigers.

This term, "canine teeth," seems to us to be somewhat imprecise because it can be used to describe the teeth of monkeys, horses, camels, lions, and dogs.

The function of these "canine" teeth in human beings is enormously different from that of actual, carnivorous canines. The same is true of their structure.

Furthermore, the long canines that monkeys possess resemble carnivorous canine teeth more than the canine teeth that humans have. However, we recognize that monkeys are vegetarians, is it not? So what? In fact, they are used not for aggressive purposes but as defensive weapons.

"If frugivores and carnivores have structural similarities," speculates Shelton, "it isn't because the former are carnivores but because the latter were initially frugivores. In fact, I think that carnivores are a deviation from first and symbiotic modes and that, in any case, this variation provoked structural and functional changes to adapt the errant animal to its inferior means of nutrition.

"However, lions would go extinct before the time came that they would peacefully cohabit with sheep or feed on grass like bulls!"

This is Shelton's response to the philosophers who have written this prophetic sentence in the Bible:

The wolf and the lamb will feed together, and the lion will eat straw like the ox, and dust will be the serpent's food. They will neither harm nor destroy on all my holy mountain," says the LORD. **Isaiah 65:25**

That is, all animals will once again become vegetarians, just as they were before when time began at the moment of creation.

Humans Are Not Herbivores

Let's return for a moment to the comparative study of species suggested in the table of comparative anatomy and physiology reproduced above.

Sometimes, I meet vegetarians who eat whole fruits, seeds and skins included. They would eat an orange with its bitter peel, or, to alleviate the bitterness, they would blend it, doing the same thing with citrus and its zest. They eat melons with both their seeds and skin intact, for example, an entire apple and grapes with both their seeds and hard peel. I have never met, on the other hand, a vegetarian who would eat cherries with their stones, at least not yet!

These vegetarians imagine that it is natural to eat the entire fruit.

However, try to chew the skin of an apple, grape or tomato. You can never turn it into a purée. What your teeth are incapable of doing, your intestines are can't.

Our sensitive stomachs cannot digest the hard parts of fruits. Only herbivores can digest the tough cellulose, yet they also prefer the tender pieces of vegetables, avoiding those which have fully matured and become hard. I once saw a donkey grazing on grass, choosing the youngest blades over the higher, older ones.

When monkeys eat peanuts, they first remove the shell and reject even the delicate skin which encases the nut. They spit out the skins and seeds of citrus, grapes, cherries. They are an example to be followed. They prefer bamboo shoots to the stems.

Primates, including humans, are not equipped to digest the hard cellulose contained in fruit skin and the tough parts of foods.

The outer leaves on cabbage are too rough to be digested. They must be cooked for twice as long as the rest of the cabbage. We should put them in the pot 15 minutes before the rest.

Cellulose And Our Intestinal Flora

It isn't a question of eliminating all cellulose from our diet. All vegetarian animals in nature eat greens. Doctors pretend that the human body is incapable of digesting this cellulose. What is this cellulose? Is it reserved for horses?

Cellulose is the pulp in carrots, greens, oranges, apples, etc. When we extract juice from fruits using a centrifuge, this separates cellulose from the juice we drink, but who decided that juice was more necessary for the body than the pulp we toss aside? Our body needs both.

In fact, this cellulose sweeps out our intestines and slows peristalsis. Otherwise, the juice passes through our system too quickly.

Cellulose is perfectly digestible when the intestines are in good health, with the help of the enzymes and bacteria found in our intestinal flora. This is why we must preserve this precious flora and avoid everything which could destroy it, such as laxatives, antibiotics, medications in general, condiments, pepper, salt, hot peppers, cheese (especially fermented cheeses) and foods which are high in protein.

Cellulose is not completely indigestible as medicine pretends it is. The intestines need only be in good health.

Ordinary enzymes which break down starches and sugars in the digestive tract can also reduce cellulose into simple sugar.

"Experience has shown," writes Shelton, "that if human beings can be in good health on diet of only fruits and various nuts, it would be even better if greens were added to be added to the diet."

However, since Shelton was mistaken about nuts, his experience was unfortunately distorted by his excessive (130 grams a day — or 4—5 ounces) consumption of these nuts. I've found that 20—30g (one ounce) can suffice and be beneficial.

Let us note in passing that gorillas do not eat nuts, that they prefer to eat nothing but fruit during the summer and nothing but greens during the winter, if the winter is harsh.

Dr. Schaller's direct observations in Africa, related in his book *The Year of the Gorilla,* and studies done at a zoological garden in San Diego, California, along with those from a Japanese zoologist have all confirmed this. We have discussed this subject many times.

In conclusion, human beings are vegetarians, capable of eating fruits, greens, and vegetables.

And to Survive?

In general, humanity has always sustained itself almost exclusively on fruits and vegetables, eaten in their natural state, since ancient times, up until very recently in human history, just before the discovery of fire.

However, while the majority of humanity was living in a tropical climate, a small group of humans was misplaced in Europe, Asia, and even the North Pole. Trapped by the cold, snow, drought and famine, humans had to turn to hunting, grains and, rarely, cannibalism to survive.

Grains were easy to store, especially during times of hardship, drought and war – at least, it was easier to store than perishable fruits and vegetables, which were rare in winter and impossible to have delivered due to the lack of adequate means of communication in those times.

Note that in nature, animals whose instinct is more intact and purer, would rather die in times of famine than eat their neighbors or children, but human beings, with our depraved instincts, were able to eat animals and even other dying humans to survive.

In short, while humans had to eat wheat and meat to survive, they paid the dear price of their health in exchange.

Humans Are Not Granivorous

In the table that we previously studied, there is no column for granivores because they are not mammals.

Granivores are animals who primarily eat grains in their raw state, such wheat, corn, etc., in addition to fruits, sprouts, and greens. These animals are mostly birds. They are granivores. They possess a grinding gizzard which humans do not possess. They pick raw grains with their beak, which they find both delicious and attractive. Humans have no beak and must cook bread in an oven at more than 230 Celsius, which strips it of all of its vitamins and living matter.

Moreover, birds eat the entire grain while humans must sieve them because they are too hard for human intestines. Bran sifting has presented unsolvable problems for dietitians. If the bran is 100% eliminated, there are no more vitamins and mineral salts. They have tried sifting it to 90—95% so that it doesn't irritate the intestines, but an ideal ratio has not been found. Moreover, it will never be seen because it doesn't exist.

Furthermore, grains contain phytic acid, which is a decalcifying agent.

In their natural state, grains are neither attractive nor appetizing for human beings like apples, pears, strawberries, and pineapples are.

Look at birds, for example. They are very attracted to the sight of grains, held out for them in your hand.

Human salivary glands secrete ptyalin to transform starch into glucose, but they only produce enough for the small amount of starch we find in foods like carrots and roots. We do not secrete enough to digest the enormous quantity of starch contained in bread and other grains.

The physiological equipment of human beings was certainly not designed to process grains. Our teeth, intestines, salivary glands, stomach and, in particular, our liver are quickly overwhelmed and exhausted by these foods.

Consuming bread and grains under these conditions leads to illnesses from the metabolic wastes that accumulate following their digestion. The time required for these diseases to develop depends on the person's age, resistance, genetics and the amount consumed.

Shelton contributed these illnesses to an excess of dairy products, but in my experience and observations, I've repeatedly found that they are due to grains. Stop eating bread, and you will stop getting colds!

Humans Are Not Carnivores

Our opposition to meat, justified by the study of the comparative anatomy and physiology of various species on earth, also applies to all other foods which are rich in proteins, whether it's meat, fish, chicken, cheese, egg whites, legumes, oysters, and shellfish.

In short, humans are not equipped to kill, tear and eat prey. They do not have claws, true canine teeth, fur or a large, powerful liver. They do not perspire through their tongue as dogs and lions do.

Meat contains a high amount of proteins. We have learned that we must only eat enough meat to obtain a sufficient quantity of protein, yet we have seen in another chapter that scientists have discovered muscular, healthy, vigorous people living from only 30 grams of protein each day. These people do not eat meat, just fruits, and vegetables which contain less than 1% protein or 3—25% for dried foods, depending on the food.

This fact is the only one that counts, and the various theories that would have us eat more meat—based proteins and other high—protein foods have no value when compared to this example taken from real life. When facts are in contradiction with theories, we must follow the facts, not the theories.

Illnesses brought on by high—protein foods by the quantity consumed are as follows:

- Infectious diseases, pus, skin disorders (eczema, psoriasis, acne), cancer, tumors.
- Mental disorders, pessimism, melancholy, agony, fear, depression, hysteria, obsession.
- Ulcers.
- Renal diseases.
- Insomnia and hypertension.

One need only stop consuming foods with high concentrations of proteins and undergo a curative fast to detoxify the body to cure the majority of mental illnesses. They don't require this trendy stupidity that we call psychoanalysis. I've successfully cared for many very advanced cases which went on to lead healthy lives like the rest of the world after years of mental distress.

When we say that 25—30% of human mortality results from cancers, we must immediately think of the excessive amounts of meat we consume. Eating meat twice daily in any form (fish, chicken, seafood) is sufficient to lay the foundation for cancer 20 years down the road. Those who consume meat only twice per week will suffer from less severe illnesses.

> **Notes from the publisher:** Again, Mosséri was ahead of his time in his observation that excess animal protein drives cancer. This is before *The China Study!*

CHAPTER 10: Testimonials

Pythagoras?

Mr. Mosséri,

As I had the opportunity to tell you during our phone conversation today, it is with great interest that I have "devoured" your latest works:

Man, Monkey, and Paradise
Antimedicine

> **Notes from publisher:** *Parts of these books were used in putting together this program.*

I find that for someone who is self—taught, you are rather "heavyweight," and there are surely very few so—called academic intellectuals who could come close to your league, and that's coming from one of those scholars!

You align yourself with Thomson and Shelton. Personally, I wouldn't hesitate to situate you next to great philosophers like Pythagoras. To find evidence of this comparison, one need only read Pythagoras' *Golden Verses* or Porphyry's *On Abstinence from Animal Food*.

May you remain a faithful servant of the truth.

My sincerest respects,

H.P.
Strasbourg

A Ray Of Sunshine

Dear Mr. Mosséri,

Your work, *Man, Monkey, and Paradise*, is a ray of sunshine, beaming from heights onto this world of shadows. Your book must be known by every truth—seeker.

Best wishes and profound peace.
L.R. – Lodeve.

In Good Shape

Mr. Mosséri,

The B family sends you our best wishes for 1992.

We are now in good shape thanks to your diet, and we have no desire to change.

Most sincerely,
M.L.B.

My Bedside Book

Dear Mr. Mosséri,

I've just read your book *Fast to Live Again*, and it has become a bedside book. I consult it all the time throughout the day, and I occasionally even read it at night. Each time, I draw from it an unexpected treasure.

> **Note from publisher:** This book has been translated as part of our program, *The Greatest Cure on Earth*.

Of all of your books, I prefer this one because it contains everything.

It has profoundly touched me. This is the first time that reading a book about food has truly satisfied me and the first time that I've said to myself that I will never have to read another.

Your book contains the truth. I feel that other authors lose themselves in the details.

Some say that tomatoes must be banned while others disagree. Some say that citrus must be banned while others disagree. Some say that eggs must be banned while others disagree.

Who should we believe? Any reader can't help but be perplexed. As a result, I think that many people become discouraged and give up following these unsuccessful attempts.

Personally, I made some deplorable mistakes during the time I spent researching.

I think it can be dangerous to decide to reform one's diet without a competent guide. It can even lead to death.

In my opinion, most authors don't follow through because they're afraid. The truth is always scary because it doesn't allow for any compromise.

I am also sometimes afraid, but I feel as though I am pushed by an unquenchable thirst for truth and perfection.

I am aware that seeking the ideal diet should be an end in itself. We must manage to surpass this stage.

All in good time!

For now, I must fight to recover my physical integrity.

I plan to do a long fast during my next summer vacation…

Anne, Dammary—Lès—lys.

Leukemia

Sir,

I have been a follower of Natural Hygiene for many years. I am a professor of physical fitness and was a medicine student (which I quit to pursue biology for personal reasons). I have studied nutrition at length, both official and naturopathic, in France and abroad. In this respect, I have often been compelled to return to theories that I was taught because it seems to me that they don't always correspond with reality.

Over the years, I taught nutrition and physical education before opening a dietary consulting office. In spite of my official diplomas, I fell, as many unfortunately do, beneath the lightning of the College. Disgusted, I converted back to agricultural science and beekeeping. I am currently in the Central African Republic for a while.

Quite a while ago I stopped eating meat in all forms. I eliminated eggs from my diet one year ago.

As for your most recent books, I must congratulate you on your works. You have done something wonderful in popularizing matters of Natural Hygiene. In these works, I recognize the profound experience of "field" technicians.

Regarding health, too many people write whatever they want, but what experience do they have? Look at what's happening with naturopathy. It's a scandal right now. No one agrees, and a new school of thought arises every day. No one wants to keep things in perspective. Everyone wants their method to be the best. Naturopaths are criticizing allopathy, but what are they doing better?

At one time, some people (and not the minority) severely criticized Shelton's food combinations, yet it's so very logical. They are currently coming back to it. None of that has much credibility and discredits the profession.

J.T. Bangui, Central African Republic

A Motorcycle Accident

Dear Mr. Mosséri,

Since my motorcycle accident on September 9th, I am doing much better. I had an open tibia fracture.

I refused to take antibiotics and anti—inflammatory medications. However, I did have a few aspirin during the first week to ease the pain. After that, I allowed nature to take its course while eating properly.

On October 11th, the cast was removed. There were no complications. The bone had healed without infection.

I am currently going through physical therapy to loosen my ankle as it has become rigid from forced immobilization.

I feel as though I'm in the clear, but all the same, I was a bit afraid. The doctors persisted and scared me so that I would agree to be poked and prodded, but I stood my ground and remained confident in nature.

I am so grateful to you, Mr. Mosséri. With the help of your books, you have guided me on the path to healthiness.

I've received your book, *Man, Monkey, and Paradise*. It is fascinating and full of insights.

Best wishes, Mr. Mosséri.
D.D. Grenoble

An Illuminating Landmark

Dear Mr. Mosséri,

I received your book, *Man, Monkey, and Paradise*, in good time, and I would like to send you my thanks.

This work is truly an illuminating landmark in the darkness which currently plagues humanity.

Unlike Nietzsche, I don't believe in a "divinely—revealed" religion (all prophets are liars). I opt for the intuitive wisdom of the great thinkers who have been betrayed by the clergy themselves.

It's hard to go against this false understanding of the world, but this work is a seed, and it will grow.

>I admire what you are fighting for and send you my warmest regards.
>M.F. Senlis

A Funtamental Book

Dear Mr. Mosséri,

I simply cannot praise your latest book, *Man, Monkey, and Paradise*, enough. Among other things, the chapter entitled "How many meals should we eat per day?" seems to me to be fundamental, totally groundbreaking and an entire program in its right, in strict accordance with the principles of Natural Hygiene. For me, it changed many of my beliefs.

I've found many great things in this book. It's very poetic, but it also goes to substantive places.

It seems to me that you are right to emphasize the manner in which fruit and water—rich vegetables are adapted to the deepest needs of the human physiology while grains, cereals, and bread are not fit for human consumption. Your way of thinking is particularly original.

The experiment seems to prove that your guidelines are correct, in particular when you distance yourself from Shelton about nuts and the pacing of meals.

Your guidelines for meal distribution and formula for "mini—meals" is entirely original, and I believe, based on my experience, that this meal plan is best for the physiology of human beings.

Thank you for this rich, well—argued, well—documented book which seems to be solid in its foundations.

You are the best Natural Hygienist I know, well above Shelton and Fry, in particular with this latest book! You have collected all the best principles of the hygienist lifestyle, those which best conform to the laws of Nature, all while taking into account their applicability.

Among these principles, I would particularly like to point out:

- Primacy and absolute respect of hunger

- The formula for "mini—meals" which opposes the firmly established institution of "meals." To my knowledge, you are the first to promote this way of eating.
- The notion of foods which are fit for human consumption, such as water—rich vegetables and fruit, as opposed to foods which are not fit for human consumption, such as grains, nuts, and legumes.

These principles are excellent, and I have only seen them combined into a single diet in your works.

Moreover, the compromises you point out — and bless you for that, for we are not saints — are the very best, in my opinion.

The whole—wheat bread trend is currently becoming popular thanks to the influence of registered dietitians who recommend "slow" carbohydrates (those which are digested slowly, they write), a category which also includes white beans, lentils, and dried peas, which are being restored to a place of honor.

Even in small villages, you can now find bakeries making whole—wheat, farmhouse and bran bread.

Out of sheer curiosity, I occasionally walk into stores which sell health and diet products. For quite some time now, I have been stunned and intrigued by the type of person that seems to frequent these shops — those buying honey, whole—wheat bread, goat cheese, camembert, etc... They don't appear to be healthy and in good shape. On the contrary, their skin is tinted gray or yellow, they're anxious and sometimes excessively thin, they're balding, and they wear dentures, indicating that they are losing their teeth. After reading your books, I now understand.

At the same time, I ask myself whether or not the effectiveness of this new method of fasting (tongue color) which you have invented is maintaining the ideal primitive conditions of fasting by only providing a minimal amount of nutrients? Doesn't it seem as though one of the major causes of poor health is too much food? In ideal primitive conditions, weren't fruits and vegetables scarce (wild fruits, for example, were much smaller and less sweet)? Isn't the absolute respect for hunger that you have so strongly emphasized often the least respected and the most difficult to maintain?

Sincerely and respectfully,
J. –L. B. Rennes.

The Book Of Books

Dear Mr. Mosséri,

First of all, allow me to thank you for your book, *Man, Monkey, and Paradise*. For me, it is the Book of Books, in the greatest possible degree. It is a leading figure in the books that I am familiar with on this subject, which is already few and far between.

You have done tremendous work, and I cannot find adequate words with which to thank you. Everything that I might say by way of praises would not capture your real worth.

I am 100% in agreement with your ideas and your writings, and I pray to God Almighty that he may bless you both in Heaven and on earth. I love you like a brother, and I thank God for giving me the opportunity to know you. I am both grateful and eternally indebted to you.

Sir, I leave you with your work, though not in thought. Thank you for much for everything that you have done in the past, the present and all that you will do in the future. May God resolve some of the difficulties you encounter with opponents of Natural Hygiene.

I send you my most respectful greetings and sincerest thanks. May God bless you and keep you in his light.

Cordially,
E.B. – Lausanne

With All My Heart

Mr. Mosséri,

I am still following a Natural Hygiene diet (that of the gorilla), and despite working as an on—site electrician doing manual labor, I am in excellent shape.

This winter, despite being in a hostile environment (surrounded by the flu, bronchitis, the common cold, and sinusitis), I didn't miss a single day of work, whereas last year, I spent a week in bed because of the flu. I owe my health this winter to eliminating grains from my diet.

This just confirms your work and your opinion on the harm that grains can inflict on the body. I alternate a meal of fruits with a meal of raw vegetables and adjust the quantity to match my hunger. Since I eat large amounts of raw vegetables at each meal (1.2 kg), I accompany them with a bit of cooked cheese as you have suggested. Someday, I hope to eliminate even this cheese from my diet.

> **Note from the publisher:** Mosseri recommended a very small amount of cheese to his French followers, as a compromise while transitioning to his diet

With all this, I rest a lot (nap or stretch out in the sun), and I go for walks. For now, everything is going well.

A year later:

I hope that my letter finds you in good health and good spirits despite the difficult challenges you are facing. I am profoundly disgusted to see that people attack and attempt to silence a man such as yourself who works so that people can rediscover their health and their true nature, two things which are at the base of all harmonious lives.

> **Note from the publisher:** Mosséri had many problems throughout his career with the medical community, including a judgement that prevented him from advertising for Natural Hygiene.

Thanks to your works on Natural Hygiene, I have rediscovered my lightness and strength. I have followed your diet for one year. 60% of my diet consists of fruits, and in the evening, the remaining 40% is raw greens and vegetables. If my hunger persists, I'll eat some cooked bananas. I eliminated nuts and cheese from my diet three months ago.

This year, I haven't experienced a single cold nor flu nor sinusitis, etc. My family has found this quite strange! What happiness I've found being freed from the drudgery of the kitchen! What time I've saved!

I owe all of this to you, Mr. Mosséri. This is why I support you with all of my heart and mind and would drive away these mercantilist, profit—oriented people who would oppose your work.

Lastly, I want to give you my thoughts on your work, *Man, Monkey, and Paradise*. It is truly a bible for Natural Hygiene practitioners and a guide in times of doubt. If there were a Nobel Prize for Health, it would be awarded to you.

I am beginning my sixth year as a lover of natural hygiene. My family gave me six months before I would start to experience severe health problems with my meals of exclusively fruits and vegetables. They didn't want to admit that it's possible for someone to live without bread, grains, cheese, meats, etc.

For two years, I didn't even see the shadow of a doctor, dentist or pharmacist.

At the moment, I am working in masonry for four hours each day. My job requires strength. The only supplement that I take is that of vegetables and fresh or dried fruits during the winter: figs, soaked raisins or dates.

I am currently experimenting with eating several small meals each day. This has proved quite difficult as we are conditioned from childhood to eat two main meals each day, but I have already succeeded in having mini—meals two days per week.

Jean Pierre T. – Balaruc Les Bains

Fit to Bear Arms

Dear Sir,

First of all, allow me to thank you for your unconditional devotion to human suffering.

Personally, the results I have seen from two years of eating fruits and vegetables have thrilled the practitioners I've consulted. Notably, an iridologist noted that I had a perfect balance of mineral salts. A psychiatric expert observed my excellent physical and mental state and deemed that I was fit to bear arms.

Jean Claude Tscheshy, Switzerland.

Note from Mossèri — This patient suffered from a severe nerve disease.

I Feel Better

Mr. Mossèri,

In spite of the worries which ail you and how overwhelmingly busy you are, you display courage, seriousness, and stoicism. I am always pleasantly surprised to receive responses from you in such a timely manner. Thank you. Without knowing it, your attitude inspires confidence. A healthy way of life corresponds with a healthy mentality. The two are intimately linked.

Personally, I have truly begun to feel better ever since I began exclusively eating fruits and vegetables and eliminating all high—protein foods. The fear of missing out has been replaced by the certainty that this was the source of my problems. Ever since my muscle and joint pain have faded away, and I have become less tense. My initial feelings of weakness have diminished. It has been replaced by a sense of well—being thanks to you and your precious works, which I read several times a day. Thank you so much.

Thank you again, and may you keep the faith, high spirits, and excellent health. You truly deserve it.

D.D. ST Leu

Made in the USA
Columbia, SC
31 March 2018